THE ULTIMATE CALISTHENICS COLLECTION

THE GYM-LESS WORKOUT + USE IT, OR LOSE IT - HOW TO MASTER BODYWEIGHT TRAINING AND TAKE IT TO THE NEXT LEVEL WITH YOUR COMPLETE GUIDE TO STRETCHING

MILO KEMP

© Copyright 2020 - All rights reserved.

The content contained within this book may not be reproduced, duplicated or transmitted without direct written permission from the author or the publisher.

Under no circumstances will any blame or legal responsibility be held against the publisher, or author, for any damages, reparation, or monetary loss due to the information contained within this book, either directly or indirectly.

Legal Notice:

This book is copyright protected. It is only for personal use. You cannot amend, distribute, sell, use, quote or paraphrase any part, or the content within this book, without the consent of the author or publisher.

Disclaimer Notice:

Please note the information contained within this document is for educational and entertainment purposes only. All effort has been executed to present accurate, up to date, reliable, complete information. No warranties of any kind are declared or implied. Readers acknowledge that the author is not engaged in the rendering of legal, financial, medical or professional advice. The content within this book has been derived from various sources. Please consult a licensed professional before attempting any techniques outlined in this book.

By reading this document, the reader agrees that under no circumstances is the author responsible for any losses, direct or indirect, that are incurred as a result of the use of the information contained within this document, including, but not limited to, errors, omissions, or inaccuracies.

CONTENTS

THE GYM-LESS WORKOUT

Introduction	7
1. Enrollment - Everything You Need to Know to Get Started	13
2. Foundations - Building up the Vital Movements	29
3. Guidance - The Routine That Will Get Results	66
4. Development - Controlling Your Own Progression	73
5. Evolution - Achieving Next-Level Movements	84
6. Evaluation - Targeting Your Weaknesses	118
7. Adaption - Mistakes You Can Avoid	170
8. Optimization - The Lifestyle You Should Aim For	187
Your mission should you choose to accept it…….	206
Conclusion	207
References	217

USE IT OR LOSE IT

Introduction	231
1. The Warm-Up: Benefits of Stretching That You Are Missing Out On	235
2. Conditioning: All the Stretches You Will Ever Need to Know	268
3. Repetitions: Stretching Routines That Make You Recover Faster	316
4. The Final Push: Stretching Routines to Optimize Your Workouts	375

5. The Cool Down: The Routine to Keep You, Young — 404
Your mission should you choose to accept it....... — 429
Conclusion — 431
References — 433

THE GYM-LESS WORKOUT

CALISTHENICS: THE BODYWEIGHT TRAINING TO CREATE RIDICULOUS PHYSIQUES WITHOUT THE GYM

<u>FREE</u> WORKOUT PLANNER & KILLER CORE WORKOUT

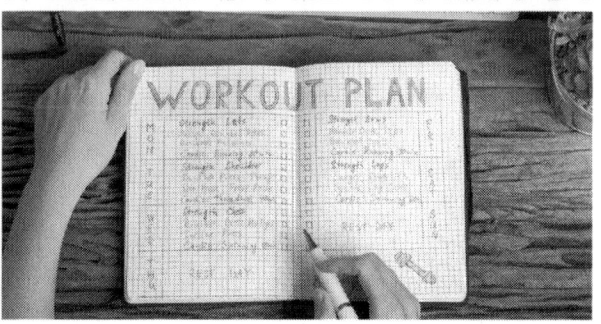

Want to make sure you reach your fitness goals?....you won't without tracking your progress! and did you know most exercises depend on a strong core for results?

1. Get your FREE perfect workout planner.
2. Get my FREE killer core workout so you reach your goals faster
3. Simply print off or download onto your device
4. And feel amazing as you watch your progress skyrocket

to receive just type in the following link :)........

https://fitnessmilo.activehosted.com/f/1

INTRODUCTION

Do you find the gym boring or intimidating? Do you have trouble finding the appeal of weightlifting? Are you tired of following the same old routines and exercises every day? You are not the only one. Countless individuals find the gym daunting or uninspiring. With all those seemingly professional athletes and exercise enthusiasts, the gym can be a very intimidating place. To put the cherry on top, carving time out of your busy schedule to travel to and from the gym can be very challenging and even demotivating. Weightlifting and machine exercises are not enjoyable experiences for everyone. What if I told you that you don't have to lift weights or use exercise machines to lose weight and build the body you want? What if I told you that you don't need any exercise equipment? What if you could be healthy and fit without even having to go to the gym? With Calisthenics, you can have the healthy, athletic body that you have always dreamed of without going to the gym, and without having to use any exercise equipment.

Calisthenics is a solution that will allow you to achieve your fitness goals with the freedom to exercise anywhere and anytime you want, all without the use of any equipment. This book will share with you the transformative power of Calisthenics, which uses only your body weight when you exercise. You will quickly progress from a helpless and uneducated fitness amateur to a professional fitness fundi with the ability and the drive to achieve your fitness - and body - goals and execute even the most intense exercises. This book will help you develop into an autonomous and effective expert in Calisthenics.

With years of experience in Calisthenics, I have taught and trained countless amateurs in the art of bodyweight training. I have helped many people in their shift from helpless beginners to seasoned athletes by developing and improving their knowledge of and performance in Calisthenics. In this book, I will provide you with the same training and information used to help these people, at a fraction of the price. You will be just as effectively equipped to change your life and achieve the body of your dreams.

INTRODUCTION

There are countless benefits to choosing Calisthenics as your exercise of choice. Not only is it absolutely free, but these exercises can be done anywhere and anytime. Calisthenic exercises reduce the chances of injury and wear-and-tear on your body significantly by removing external pressure and weight. Your travel time will be reduced, leaving you with more time to invest elsewhere. Calisthenics focuses on developing movement, strength, and aesthetic, leaving you more confident than ever and giving you complete control over your body. In this book, I will share with you all that I have learned and observed over the years. In doing so, I will save you from making the same mistakes made by myself and others in the Calisthenics field. I will give you all the tools and steps that you need to start your journey in Calisthenics so that you won't have to waste any time figuring it out for yourself.

People often come to me not being able to do a single pull up and barely able to do any push-ups. Once I have worked my magic, these people can do these and much more extensive and complicated exercises. They leave enlightened and inspired to take control of their bodies, and you will too! In the few chapters of this book, I will guide you on your way to mastering Calisthenics. Like these people, you will be able to do exercises ranging from basic movements to the most complicated, extensive, and muscle-taxing exercises.

INTRODUCTION

In this book, I will give you all the tools you need to start your journey. I will provide you with a basic understanding of Calisthenics and what it entails, including the benefits of Calisthenics and what makes this kind of exercise more effective than other conventional exercise methods such as weightlifting. I will then take you through the most basic movements of Calisthenics and provide you with steps on how to do these movements, including further variations of each of these movements and exercises. I will give you everything you need to know to establish an effective routine that will guarantee results. I will provide some guidance on determining the level at which to start and how to control and master your own progression. I will also share with you some exercise strategies to achieve the most complicated and taxing movements, such as the human flag and the 90-degree push-up. I will discuss the difference between split and full-body workouts, and I will provide you with some examples of split workouts. I will also explain some of the most common mistakes and injuries in Calisthenics, and how these can be avoided or rectified. Finally, I will provide you with some guidance on how to create a conducive lifestyle that will support your goals and help you achieve the desired results by focusing on diet, sleeping patterns, consistency, and on building healthy habits.

After reading this book, you will be able to manage your own exercise routine efficiently and control your own progressions. This book will leave you with the skills and the mindset that you need to achieve your desired transformation. You will have a better understanding of what Calisthenics is and what it entails. You will be equipped to maintain the correct form in your exercises and avoid the most common mistakes and injuries. At the end of this book, you should be able to build a healthy lifestyle that accommodates your newfound skills and passion for Calisthenics. By applying the knowledge and skills discussed in this book, you will be able to improve your physique and achieve the body you desire in no time.

Reading this book is only the beginning, however. The real work starts once you have finished reading the book, when you are ready to begin your first bodyweight workout. Merely reading this book will not be sufficient. You will have to put in the bulk of the work yourself by applying the skills and knowledge you have learned from this book to achieve your goals and aims. Just having the knowledge and skills will not help you achieve your goals. You have to apply these strategies consistently and effectively in order to reach your desired physique. You will need to foster self-discipline, determination, and lots of patience to achieve the desired results. The first few weeks will not be easy, but it will most definitely be worth it in the long haul.

I will bring you all the knowledge, skills, and strategies you need to achieve the physique you so desperately desire. If you commit and apply these strategies and skills consistently and efficiently, you will start to see results in no time. You will soon achieve the body you desire, but the responsibility is yours to take up. Are you up for the challenge?

1

ENROLLMENT - EVERYTHING YOU NEED TO KNOW TO GET STARTED

You have taken the first steps to becoming a Calisthenics expert by purchasing this book. You may be asking yourself what Calisthenics actually is. How does muscle-building work, and what is the difference between weightlifting and bodyweight training? Before you start practicing Calisthenics or attempt any insane exercises, you will need to develop an understanding of what Calisthenics is and what the benefits of this practice are. It is also important to understand the foundational science behind muscle-building and strength. Malcolm X (AZ Quotes, n.d.) said that "Education is the passport to the future," so grab your ticket and let us dive in.

What Is Calisthenics?

Calisthenics is a form of resistance training that uses only body weight. It requires no additional weights or equipment. Rather, it relies solely on the natural weight of the body. Calisthenics focuses mainly on developing movement, strength, and aesthetics. Through mindful exercise and controlled movement, it improves various aspects of bodily function, including strength, endurance, flexibility, agility, balance, coordination, and cardiovascular functioning. The word Calisthenics stems from two Greek words: *Kalos* meaning 'beauty' and *stenos* meaning 'strength.' The Greek origin, therefore, focuses on the strength and aesthetic nature of bodyweight training.

Warming up before a workout and cooling down post-workout are very important phases of any exercise. Warm-ups get your blood flowing and warm up the muscles. Warmer muscles respond better to challenging and straining exercises and significantly reduce the chances of injury, sprains, or pains. Cardiovascular exercises are the most effective option for pre-workout warm-ups. Coming to an abrupt stop after your exercise can make you feel light-headed and dizzy. Cool-down exercises prevent your heart rate and blood pressure from dropping too rapidly and therefore reduce the chances of experiencing light-headedness and dizziness. Stretches and mild cardiovascular exercises are best for cooling down after a workout.

There are a number of other things that you need to take

THE GYM-LESS WORKOUT

note of regarding Calisthenics. These are crucially important to keep in mind while you practice.

1. Having the correct form during exercises is a key aspect of Calisthenics. Executing exercises with the wrong form can cause unnecessary injury and may, in some cases, render the exercise useless. Having the correct form during an exercise helps the body to engage the necessary muscles to produce optimal results.
2. It is also essential to focus your mind on the task or exercise at hand. One of the benefits of Calisthenics is that it improves the brain-body connection. This can only be achieved effectively if the mind is focused on the exercise at hand.
3. In Calisthenic exercises, quality is significantly more important than quantity. Doing a larger number of reps of an exercise is useless if your form is not correct. Instead, do fewer reps and focus on achieving the perfect form. This will produce better results than doing more reps with inconsistent or incorrect form.
4. Breathing is another important aspect to pay attention to. Inhale when contracting and exhale when expanding. This helps you to execute

exercises more efficiently and will also assist with focus during the exercise.

If you are a beginner Calisthenic, start with the most basic variations of exercises and use progressions to improve yourself. Basic exercises and progressions will be discussed in Chapter 2 of this book.

The Science of Muscle-Building

Now that you understand what Calisthenics is and what aspects to pay attention to let me give you a simplified breakdown of the physiology of strength- and muscle-building. The process of muscular growth is essentially a cycle of damaging and repairing muscle tissue. The kind of exercises you do will determine the types of adaptations and changes that take place in your muscular structure. When we train or exercise, we cause muscle damage and cause the muscle tissue to break down. This forces the muscles to restructure themselves and grow back bigger and stronger than before. When we experience muscle damage, satellite cells move in to repair the damage that was caused by fusing muscle fibers and forming new muscle protein strands. Over time, these strands get thicker and increase in number, leading to muscle growth. If the rate of repair is greater than the rate of muscle damage, muscle growth occurs.

It is important to note, however, that muscle growth technically occurs during periods of rest. It is during periods of rest and sleep that these satellite cells can move in and repair the muscle damage. Therefore, not getting enough rest will put your body into a destructive state. Your damage-to-repair ratio will be imbalanced, and your body will not have enough time to recover, leaving your muscles in a semi-permanently damaged state. The process of muscle regrowth will only be successful if you provide your body with enough rest, and with the nutrients it needs to repair the muscle damage. That is why sleep and nutrition are essential parts of an active lifestyle. The effects of diet and nutrition will be discussed in further detail in Chapter 8. Muscle growth is a slow process and may take weeks or even months before it becomes visible. Patience is a virtue, but in time, you will most definitely reap the hard-earned rewards of your hard work.

BENEFITS OF CALISTHENICS

Now that you know what Calisthenics is, the next step is to consider why you should choose Calisthenics as your exercise strategy of choice. Calisthenics is an innovative and sustainable solution for a number of reasons. There are countless benefits to choosing Calisthenics as your exercise strategy. Consider the following benefits:

Calisthenics is for anyone.

With its various levels of progression and all its variations, Calisthenics is an appropriate strategy for anyone and everyone, ranging from beginners to experts. Regressions and variations allow for beginners to focus on their form with easier variations of basic exercises. These exercises will build the necessary foundations and can then be adapted as needed to support progress and growth. For professional athletes and fitness experts, there are countless more complex variations to consider, which can make these exercises more challenging, interesting, and a lot more fun.

Calisthenics can be done anywhere, anytime!

Calisthenics focuses solely on the use of body weight. This means that you can do these exercises anywhere and at any time. You can use the monkey bars in the park for your pull-up exercises or your bedroom floor for sit-ups. You can even do calf raises in your chair behind your desk at work. The possibilities are endless. Calisthenics is the perfect solution for busybodies and workaholics.

Practicing Calisthenics is virtually free.

Did I mention that Calisthenics can be done anywhere? This means that you need not pay hefty gym membership fees any longer. With absolutely no cost involved, Calisthenics is definitely a sustainable solution.

No equipment needed.

If you just don't see the appeal of weightlifting, don't worry. Although weight can be added to improve progress and complicate exercises, Calisthenics requires no additional equipment or weights. Some equipment, such as chairs, stools, or boxes, can be found in most homes, while others, such as horizontal or vertical bars, can easily be found in outdoor places such as parks. If you do want to attempt exercises such as weighted pull-ups, a loaded backpack can be just as efficient as a weighted belt or vest.

Calisthenics keeps exercise interesting.

Calisthenics is one of the most interesting and exciting forms of exercise. Most exercises, like weightlifting, require repetitive and set routines, and there aren't many alternatives. Many forms of exercise are limited in terms of the range of available exercises, and progressions can only be made by adding more weight. Calisthenics offers a wide variety of exercises, and there are countless variations and progressions (or regressions) for these exercises. There are hundreds of options to choose from. Forget about the same old boring routines. Calisthenics keeps exercise new, exciting, and innovative. Since you can do these exercises anywhere, you can't even get bored with your exercise space. Changing things up adds new excitement and flavor to life and exercise.

Quicker rest and recovery rates.

With heavy exercises such as weightlifting, rest, and recovery can take a while. With Calisthenics, however, this is not the case. Since Calisthenics reduces the external load and strain on your body, rest and recovery rates are much quicker, making this an efficient option. Shorter rest and recovery rates also make Calisthenics much more effective at burning fat.

Progression is easy!

Progression is not a problem when it comes to Calisthenics. With innumerable variations and progression strategies, exercises can easily be personalized and adapted to suit your needs. Amateurs and professionals alike can easily plan and implement strategies for the progression or regression of exercises tailored to their skill level and ability.

Calisthenics improves weightlifting abilities.

Calisthenics improves your core strength and gives you more control over your body, making weightlifting much easier and more manageable. Practicing Calisthenics can significantly improve your weightlifting techniques and capabilities. It helps you to develop the fundamental skills to perform the most basic exercises with perfect form. This skill will help you avoid unnecessary injury and ease the training process significantly.

Improved self-confidence.

Calisthenics not only helps you look good but will also help you feel good. The level of progression and improvement in your body's aesthetic will leave you feeling more confident than ever. The knowledge that you can do these exercises is also a contributing factor. Who wouldn't want to feel good about themselves?

Calisthenics improves the brain-body connection.

While machine and weight training focuses on training your body muscles, Calisthenics improves both body and brainpower. Calisthenic exercises require focus and engage your mind. Maintaining the correct form requires not only bodily strength but also brainpower. By enhancing your brain-body connection, your body's reaction time will also be improved significantly, leaving you sharper and healthier than ever.

Calisthenics is gentler on your joints and connective tissue.

Since Calisthenics focuses solely on using bodyweight, it places no additional weight and strain on your joints. People who add heavy weights during their exercises can experience joint pains and injuries. This occurs because the additional weight puts extra strain on their muscles and connective tissue. Using only your body weight during exercise will reduce the risk of joint pains and injury.

Train every single muscle.

Most Calisthenic exercises focus on multiple muscles simultaneously. It, therefore, helps you to exercise all your muscles more efficiently and offers an all-round improvement, instead of focusing on one muscle at a time.

Maintain better form.

Calisthenic exercises make it more possible to focus on form when exercising. Since Calisthenics removes most of the strain and offers more variations and easier progressions, it is easier to focus on maintaining the correct form, which will inevitably help you produce better results. As will be discussed throughout the course of the book, progressions can help you to develop and maintain the correct form when exercising, making the exercises more effective and preventing unnecessary injury and strain.

Improve your functional strength to help you move better in real life.

Calisthenics helps you to build balance and prevents injury in various ways. Being more in control of your body and reducing joint pains and injury will help you to move better and more functionally in your day-to-day engagements.

Calisthenics will leave you feeling better all-round. Core exercises are known for improving posture. Since Calisthenics focuses heavily on building core strength, it will help you to improve your posture as an added bonus. Its tendency to improve brain-body coordination will also help you to improve your body's reaction time significantly. You will be able to act and react at a much quicker pace.

Calisthenics builds strength.

Since Calisthenics works multiple muscles simultaneously, it helps build strength more quickly and efficiently. Calisthenics focuses not only on building strength in certain muscles but gives you an all-round improvement in full-body strength. By developing and strengthening a range of muscles, Calisthenics will allow you to do exercises that defy gravity and seem to break the laws of Physics.

Calisthenic exercises are efficient.

Doing Calisthenics requires no gym and no equipment. You don't need to drive to and from the gym or spend time loading or unloading weights onto your equipment. What's more, by focusing on several muscles simultaneously, you get to spend more time exercising more muscles for better results. Doing Calisthenics will save you a lot of time and effort and allow you to achieve more in the time you do exercise.

Get rid of body fat.

Since Calisthenics trains multiple muscles at a time, it is very efficient for burning body fat. By applying shorter rest periods between sets, you enable your body to burn fat faster and more efficiently. This approach is known as metabolic resistance training.

Calisthenics strengthens your core and unloads your spine.

Calisthenic exercises focus significantly on improving core strength. Most Calisthenic exercises involve the core in some way. By not involving extra or excessive weight, Calisthenics is generally much gentler on the spine than weightlifting exercises. Some exercises like planks focus on strengthening your spine, and Calisthenic exercises, in general, help improve core strength without placing unnecessary pressure on your spine. Inevitably, this will also significantly reduce the chances of back and spine injuries.

Calisthenics builds a perfectly proportionate physique.

Since Calisthenics focuses on multiple muscles simultaneously, it helps to sculpt a symmetrical and proportionate physique. Unlike with other exercises, you need not worry too much about carefully balancing exercises to avoid a disproportionate physique. Calisthenics helps you to build an all-round aesthetic body and leaves you perfectly proportionate.

With all these benefits and more, it is evident that Calisthenics is an innovative and effective exercise strategy to choose.

CALISTHENICS VS. WEIGHTLIFTING

You may wonder what the difference is between weightlifting and Calisthenics. How do I know which is the better option? Both Calisthenics and weightlifting focus on building strength, but there are a number of differences between these exercises. I've touched on some of the differences already in the previous section. Still, this section will make an all-round comprehensive comparison between Calisthenics and weightlifting to help you decide which of these options is better suited to your needs and goals.

Weightlifting

Weightlifting is a form of resistance training that involves the use of weights and equipment to improve and build strength and endurance. Starting with weight training is often quite easy, but the results are not easy to maintain from home. Unless you have a fully equipped gym at home, weightlifting requires you to be a member and regular visitor at a gym. You might even need access to a trainer if you are unfamiliar with the dynamics of weightlifting. Access is, therefore, a key factor in weight training. Furthermore, maintaining a regular routine is very important with weight training, as missing a session can seriously affect your results as you likely will not train that muscle group again that week. Results are often directly dependent on routine and discipline. Weightlifting is, therefore, quite time-consuming and demanding.

Weightlifting is a good option for maintaining and strengthening specific muscles or muscle groups. Weightlifting exercises often isolate certain muscles or muscle groups, making it a better option if you're looking to develop specific muscles. However, this can also be done with Calisthenics, as I mention later in chapter 6. Weight training focuses on developing your maximum strength. It has a lower impact on motor reflexes, however, as it relies mostly on brute force and strength. Weightlifting is a good option if you are aiming to increase your body mass since it allows you to add more weight than your bodyweight. Weightlifting also makes it significantly easier to track your progress. All you need to do is look at the weight added to your exercises; this will help keep you motivated when the going gets tough.

Calisthenics

Calisthenics is a form of resistance training that focuses on using body weight to improve strength and flexibility. Whereas weightlifting requires a gym and the use of equipment, Calisthenics requires no equipment and can be done anywhere and at any time. It is effortless to start Calisthenics since countless variations and progressions can be applied to simplify or complicate exercises according to your needs. Beginners can use easier progressions to focus on maintaining the correct form before they delve into the more complex and progressive exercises and variations. Calisthenic exercises are better for developing endurance, as they focus mainly on shorter rest periods. Calisthenic exercises are not aimed at exercising to the point of exhaustion, but rather focus on building core strength. Due to the nature and load of Calisthenics, recovery time is often much quicker than in other exercises.

Calisthenics builds total-body strength, as it focuses on various groups of muscles at the same time, whereas weight training often focuses on strengthening one muscle or group of muscles at a time. It focuses on building relative strength - that is, how strong you are relative to your body weight, and increases the body's core strength. Calisthenics also engages the brain's motor reflexes, decreasing your reaction time and improving brain-body communication. Calisthenics is an effective weight loss solution. While weightlifting can promote weight loss, Calisthenics does so effectively and quickly. The flexibility of Calisthenic exercises allows you to adapt your schedule easily, and by decreasing rest time, you can help your body to burn more fat at a much quicker pace as you keep your heart rate higher.

Depending on your goals, Calisthenics can be better for building body mass than weightlifting. Whereas weightlifting is efficient at building specific parts of the body more rapidly, Calisthenics' tendency to focus on numerous muscles simultaneously makes it the better option for all-round body mass building. Therefore, if your goal is to develop specific muscles rapidly, weightlifting would be the better solution. To build general body mass, however, Calisthenics might be more efficient. With Calisthenics training, progress is often more difficult to track as there is no quantitative measure that indicates progress. Exercises do get easier with time, however, and can be adapted to become more difficult and challenging. Although it is harder to track progress immediately, the long-term effects of Calisthenics are definitely worth the wait.

There are a number of similarities between weightlifting and Calisthenics, and each of these has its place. You need to determine what you aim to achieve and make your decision based on that. Weightlifting would be the better option for those who want to focus on building specific muscles. For an all-round improvement and physique, however, Calisthenics is the more effective option.

2

FOUNDATIONS - BUILDING UP THE VITAL MOVEMENTS

Before jumping into the more complex and intricate Calisthenic exercises, it is essential to understand and master the basic movements of Calisthenics first. Calisthenics can broadly be broken down into four main categories: pull exercises, push exercises, leg exercises, and core exercises. Once you have mastered the basic exercises and you can execute them using the correct form, you can then move on to other variations of these exercises and other, more complex exercises. If these basic movements are too difficult, you can try the more straightforward progressions and work your way up from there. It is important to note that these exercises are but a drop in the ocean of Calisthenic exercises and variations that can be done. These are merely the foundation. Once you've managed to master these exercises, the sky is the limit.

Mastering these basic movements first is extremely important. These movements are the building blocks for most other Calisthenic movements. Being able to learn these movements will make the mastery of other, more progressive exercises easier and less taxing. Mastering the basic exercises will lay the foundation for all other exercises that you will perform and help you to execute the correct form and control that you need to complete these exercises.

PULL EXERCISES

Pull-ups

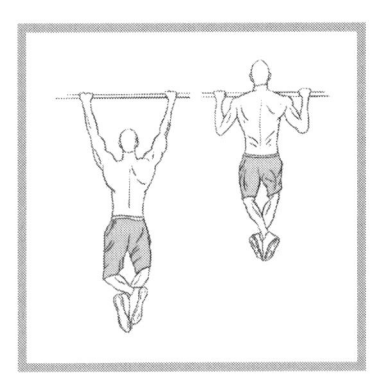

The most basic of the pull movements is the pull-up. Pull-ups focus mainly on your back, arm, and core muscles. To execute the pull-up, you will need access to a pull-up bar. This is a horizontal bar, raised about an arm's length above your head. The pull-up can be executed in four easy steps.

- Stand facing the pull-up bar.
- Grasp the bar with your hands, slightly overgrip, keeping your arms slightly more than shoulder-width apart.
- Pull yourself up towards your chest using your shoulder muscles and engaging your scapula (shoulder blades), raising your head above the bar.
- Then, lower yourself slowly using your arms and core.

In order to execute the pull-up effectively, there are several things you need to take note of.

Firstly, hold the bar at the base of your fingers instead of your palms. Doing so will prevent unnecessary wrist and arm injuries and improve your strength significantly. Keep your wrists aligned with your forearms during the exercise. Focus on your core movements to stabilize your body during the exercise. Ignoring your core movements might cause your body to swing and will result in loss of control and possible injury. Focusing on your core during the exercise, will also ensure that you work on your core muscles along with your back muscles. Lastly, it is important that you not rush the exercise. Focus on your form and execution rather than on how quickly you can do the exercise or how many you can do. Remember that quality is more important than quantity.

Progressions

Pull-ups may be tough for those who are just starting on their Calisthenic journey. Don't let this discourage you. If the pull-up is too difficult for you, there are easier variations that you can start with. If you have trouble executing a pull-up, start with Australian pull-ups. Once you are comfortable with these, you can progress to jumping pull-ups, assisted pull-ups, and finally attempt a full-on pull-up.

Australian Pull-Ups

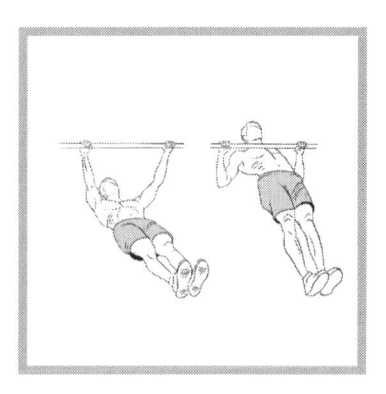

An Australian pull-up requires a lower vertical bar than the pull-up, about hip-height.

- Start by gripping the bar with your hands and lowering your body under the bar at an angle. The higher the angle of your body, the easier the exercise will be.
- Start with your arms and legs extended and pull your body toward the bar using your arms. Keep your legs extended during the exercise.
- Once you've pulled your body to the bar, lower your body slowly back to the starting position using your arms.

If you've started the exercise with a higher body angle, try to lower the angle as you progress before moving on to the next progression.

Jumping Pull-Ups

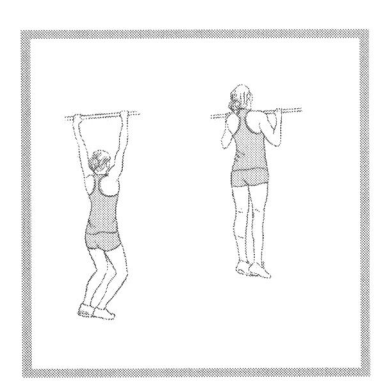

Jumping pull-ups are similar to regular pull-ups, but slightly easier. This exercise will significantly improve your arm strength and allow you to focus on lowering yourself from the extended position. To perform this exercise, you will need a pull-up bar.

- Stand facing the vertical bar.
- Grasp the bar with your hands, keeping your arms slightly more than shoulder-width apart.
- Jump up into the elevated pull-up position. Lower yourself slowly using your arms and core and let go once you have lowered your body entirely.

Once you can perform these comfortably and effectively, you can move on to the next progression.

Assisted Pull-Ups

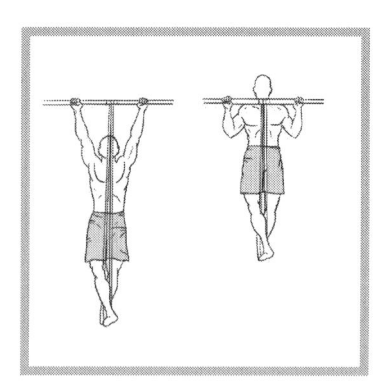

For this exercise, you will need a resistance band. This exercise is similar to regular pull-ups, but with some assistance. Fasten a resistance band onto the pull-up bar and place either one foot or both feet inside the pull-up band. Proceed to execute a pull-up with your foot or feet inside the resistance band. The resistance band will offer some support and make the pull-up movement easier to complete. Once you can achieve this exercise with ease, you can move on to attempt the pull-up.

Variations

If pull-ups seem too easy or dull, there are more complex variations that you can try. Before you attempt the more complex variations, make sure that you are able to do at least 10 pull-ups correctly and with perfect form. Once you can do a pull-up successfully and effectively, you can then move on to weighted pull-ups.

Weighted Pull-Ups

Weighted pull-ups are done using the same steps as regular pull-ups but with added weight. Weight can be added using either a weighted vest or adding a weight around your waist. If these are not accessible to you, putting a loaded backpack on your back or chest will also suffice.

Explosive pull-ups

An explosive pull-ups is what it sounds like; you want to try and complete your pull-ups with as much power as you can on the way up and then lower yourself as usual. This is also a great way to raise your heart rate higher if you aim to burn more fat or have a more intense workout.

L-sit pull-ups

A minor change to regular pull-ups by bringing your legs up to parallel to the ground creating an 'L' position; this will activate your core muscles much more than a usual pull up. It can be a beneficial exercise when looking to develop advanced movements such as the front lever and muscle up.

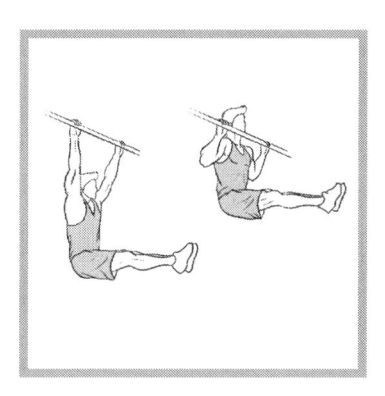

Archer pull-ups

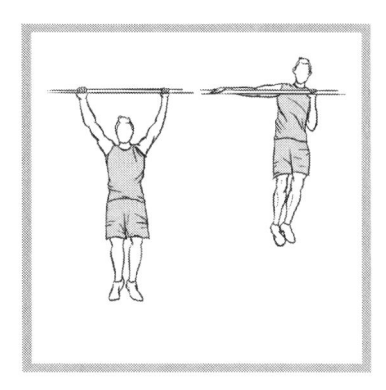

An interesting variation of the pull-up, the archer, pull up requires you to keep one arm straight while the other arm continues the action of the pull-up, naturally, this brings your torso over to the side of your bend arm. As you bring your body to the bar, your body from behind should resemble an archer about to fire an arrow.

PUSH EXERCISES

Push movements mainly focus on the chest and shoulder muscles, as well as the triceps. Most push exercises engage the abs and strengthen the core as well. The most basic of the push exercises are push-ups and dips.

Push-Ups

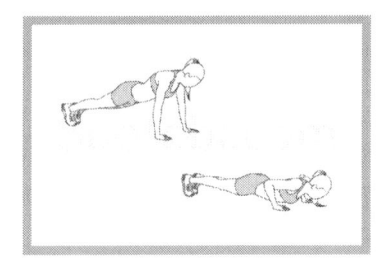

Push-ups mostly focus on strengthening the chest and arm muscles but engage the core as well. They are significantly easier than pull-ups and, similarly, have a number of variations and progressions that can be applied. There are four steps to executing a push-up.

- Position yourself on the floor on all fours. Position your hands slightly more than shoulder-width apart.
- Extend your legs backward in such a way that you are balanced on your hands and your toes. Keep your body straight - don't raise or lower your back.
- Bend your elbows and lower yourself toward the floor using your arms, keeping your elbows tucked in and triceps parallel to your torso until your chest almost touches the floor.
- Raise yourself again by pressing up with your arms until you reach your starting position. Your back should remain straight throughout the entire exercise.

There are several common mistakes that people often make when doing push-ups. Take note of these errors and keep them in mind while you exercise so that you can avoid them.

Firstly, beware of sagging (or raising) your middle while doing a push-up. Sagging your middle can cause back pain and will not produce effective results. To prevent this from happening, keep your core and torso stiff and your back straight throughout the exercise. Furthermore, your neck should be aligned with your spine, and your eyes should be focused on the floor. Do not drop or lift your head too much, as this affects your body's alignment when performing the exercise. When you come back to the starting position, do not lock your elbows. Locking your elbows can put unnecessary strain on your joints and can cause injury. Keep your elbows slightly bent at all times and tucked in; do not let them stick out perpendicular to your torso. Keep your hands directly under your shoulders. Placing your hands too far forward puts too much strain on your shoulders. Lastly, make sure that you go down as far as possible. By going down only partially, you will not reap the full benefits of the exercise.

Progressions

If doing a regular push-up is too difficult, start with some of the easier variations and move your way up. You may want to start with a bent knee push-up and proceed to an incline knee push-up and high to low plank before you face regular push-ups.

Bent Knee Push-Ups

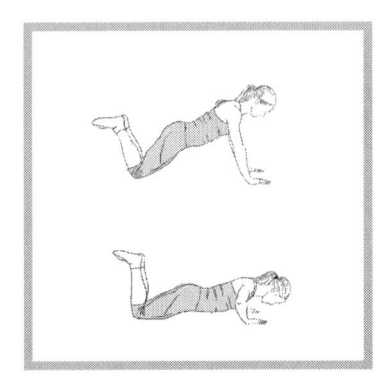

Bent knee push-ups are performed similarly to regular push-ups, with the exception that they are performed on the knees instead of the toes.

- Position yourself on the floor on all fours. Position your hands slightly more than shoulder-width apart.
- Cross your legs in the air with your knees on the floor. You should be balanced on your hands and knees only. Keep your back straight during the exercise.
- Lean your body forward, bend your elbows, and

lower yourself toward the floor using your arms until your chest almost touches the floor.
- Raise yourself up again by pressing up with your arms until you reach your starting position. Your back should remain straight throughout the entire exercise.

You should be able to do at least ten repetitions of this exercise before you move on to the next progression.

Incline Push-Ups

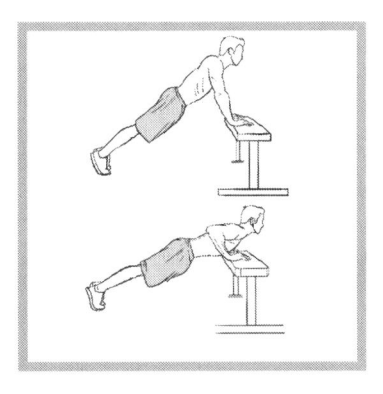

This exercise is similar to a regular push-up but is done at an incline. To do this exercise, you will need a chair, bench, or box. Anything that will help you elevate your upper body.

- Position yourself with your hands on the box and

your feet on the floor. Your arms should be extended in front of you, and you should be on your toes with your legs extended backward on the floor.
- Proceed with the same push-up movement, only at an incline this time. Make sure to keep your back straight throughout the exercise.

The steeper the incline, the easier the exercise will be. Start with a higher incline and decrease the incline as you progress. Once you are able to complete at least ten repetitions at a lower incline with perfect form, you may move onto the next progression.

High to Low Plank

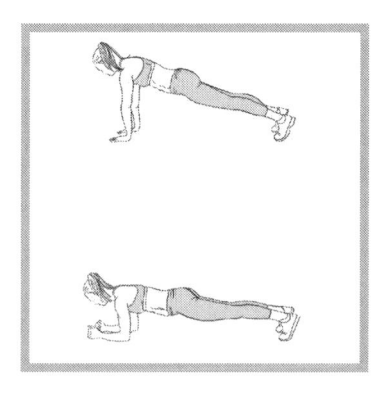

This exercise focuses mainly on strengthening your core but will also strengthen your bicep muscles.

- Start in the push-up position with your arms extended in front of you, your body raised, and your legs extended back.
- Keeping your back straight and your legs extended, lower yourself first onto one elbow, then onto the other.
- Once you have successfully moved into the plank position, proceed to extend one arm, then the other, into the starting position.

It is important that you keep your body straight and your core tight throughout this exercise. Once you can execute these perfectly and comfortably, you may proceed to attempt the push-up.

Variations

There are several very complex variations to the push-up. However, since these variations exceed the basic exercises and foundations that we are trying to develop, for now, focus on mastering the push-up with perfect form and execution.

Decline push up

Like the incline push up, you will need a chair, bench, or box to complete this push-up. Place your feet on the raised surface and lower your chest to the floor and back up again.

The height of the raised surface will correlate to the difficulty of the push-up, so to make the push up harder, use a table or taller box. Also note that a steeper angle will work your upper chest, this may be important to remember later when aiming for that well-rounded physique.

Pike push up

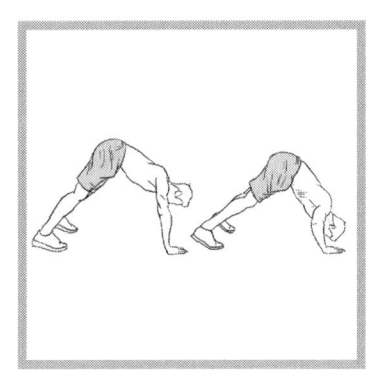

Get yourself into the position of the downwards facing dog, a popular yoga pose. Proceed to bend at the elbows lowering your crown slowly to the floor. The angle of the bend your legs make with your torso will determine the difficulty of the push up as the more acute this angle is, the stronger the force of gravity on your shoulders as you lower your crown. This variation of push-up is an excellent workout for your shoulders.

. . .

Diamond push up

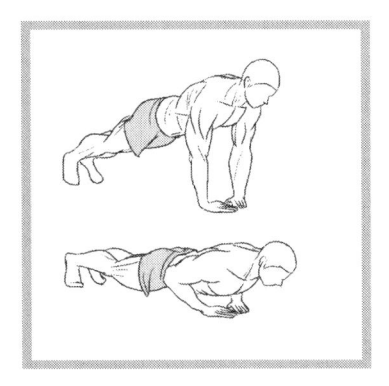

This variation of push up works your inner chest by placing your palms on the floor next to each other together, forming a triangle with your thumb and index fingers; this is the perfect hand placement. Then lower yourself to the ground and raise yourself again. It may feel unnatural and awkward at first, you can slightly adjust your hand position to see if it feels more comfortable, but you will soon get used to it.

Most variations of push up are designed to work different parts of the chest and shoulders, so including multiple of these in an upper body work will serve you well when building a well-proportioned body.

DIPS

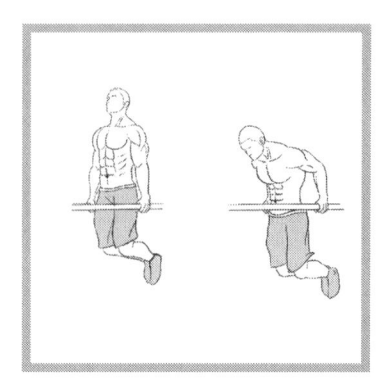

Dips target the upper body, including the abdominal, arm, and back muscles. To perform this exercise, you will need a dip bar. A dip bar consists of two waist-height parallel bars just over shoulder-width apart. If you do not have access to a dip bar, you can create a makeshift one by placing two chairs on either side of your body, just over shoulder-width apart.

- Grasp the two parallel bars (or chairs) on either side of your body with your hands shoulder-width apart.
- Raise your feet off the ground with only your arms to support your weight. Keep your knees slightly bent backward and legs crossed. Keep your elbows slightly bent at all times.

- Lower yourself by bending your elbows until your arms are at a 90-degree angle.
- Now, use your arms to push yourself up toward the starting position.

There are some common mistakes that you need to be conscious of when performing dips. Being aware of these mistakes will help you achieve perfect form and execute your dips more effectively.

Like the push-up, you should not lock your elbows at any time during the exercise. Keep your arms slightly bent at all times. Locking your elbows will require extra strength and may cause unnecessary strain or injury. Keep yourself steady; do not swing during the exercise as this may lead to injury. Do the exercise slowly and mindfully to make sure that you are using the correct form and execution. When you descend, make sure that you go down far enough, bending your elbow to a 90-degree angle. Not going down far enough will limit the potential of the exercise. Focus on your execution and form before attempting to do more dips.

Progressions

If dips are too much for you, you might try practicing some bench dips first. Once you have mastered the bench dips, you can move on to negative dips, assisted dips, and eventually move on to practicing the standard dip.

Bench Dips

Bench dips focus on strengthening your arm and shoulder muscles without the strain of your full body weight.

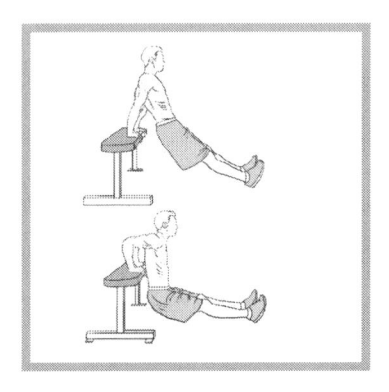

- Place a bench behind your back and place your hands on the bench about shoulder-width apart. Extend your legs in front of you and bend forward at the waist.
- Lower your body using your arms, bending your elbows to around 90 degrees. Keep your legs straight during the exercise.
- Use your triceps to lift yourself back into the starting position.

This exercise can be simplified by placing your legs at a 90-degree angle rather than extending them out straight. If you opted for the 90-degree leg angle, be sure to practice the extended leg variation before moving on to the next progression. You should be able to do at least ten of these with perfect form before moving on.

Negative Dips

Negative dips use the same principle as jumping pull-ups. They focus on isolating and developing the descending movement (eccentric) of the dip to help you both master the movement and strengthen your arm muscles.

- Grasp the two parallel bars on either side of your body with your hands shoulder-width apart.
- Instead of raising yourself, jump to the elevated position and focus on lowering yourself slow and controlled using your arms.
- Proceed to the starting position and try again.

Once you can do at least ten of these confidently, you can move to the next progression.

Assisted Dips

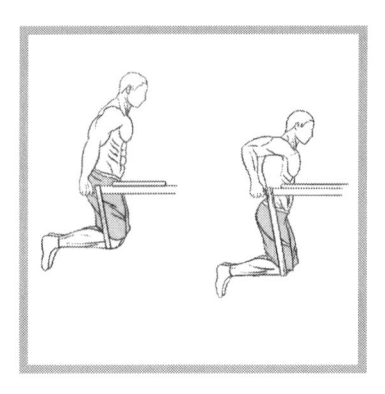

Assisted dips are based on the same principle as assisted pull-ups. You will need a resistance band to execute this exercise. By using resistance bands, you are simplifying the movements of the dip significantly while still conditioning your body to execute the movement. By taking off some of the weight, this exercise allows you to focus on the movement of the dip, paying particular attention to form and execution.

- Tie the resistance band to either side of the dip bar, place your knees inside of the resistance band in the dip position.
- Perform the same steps described for the dip, keeping your knees inside the resistance band.

When you can perform ten of these with precision, you may then proceed to the dip.

Variations

Once you have successfully mastered basic dips, you can then move on to weighted dips. You should be able to execute at least fifteen to twenty dips with precision before attempting the weighted dip.

Weighted Dips

Weighted dips follow the same steps as regular dips, but with added weight. To perform this exercise, you will need a weighted vest or weighted belt. If these are not at your disposal, you can use a loaded backpack as an alternative.

- Attach the weighted belt or weighted vest to your body.
- Proceed to perform a dip as described previously.

Even with the added weight, weighted dips should be performed with precision and attention to their execution.

L-sit dips

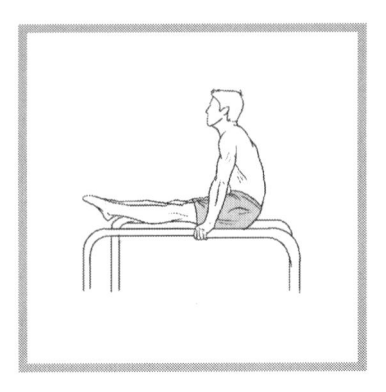

L-sit dips aim to activate your core more than a regular dip; this will add an extra dimension as you learn to control multiple muscle groups. Bring your legs up parallel to the floor and proceed to complete a dip. To make this variation easier, bring your legs into the tuck position then try extending one leg as a progression for the L-sit dip.

LEG EXERCISES

Squats

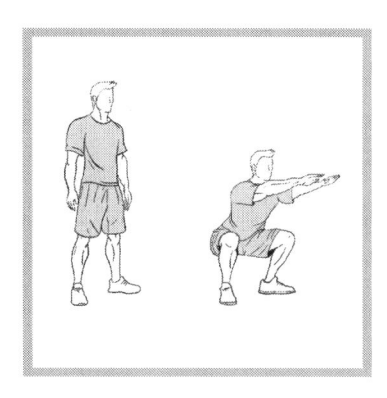

The most common and basic leg exercises are squats. Squats generally work on your legs and glutes, but can also activate several other muscles.

- Stand with your feet approximately shoulder-width apart and your toes pointing outwards.
- Lean your hips backward, bend your legs toward the floor, and move into a sitting position. Keep your chest up and shift your weight to your heels.
- Pause with your knees over your toes and your legs parallel to the floor. Do not move your knees beyond your toes.
- Using your legs, push yourself back into the starting position.

There are some things that you need to pay attention to

when doing squats. These tips will help you to execute the squat more effectively and avoid unnecessary mistakes.

The first mistake that people often make is that they try to focus the exercise on their knees. This places unnecessary strain on your knee joints and may cause injury. Instead of focusing on bending your knees, focus on moving your hips backward and think of a sitting motion. If this seems to be a challenge for you, practice this movement with a chair. Another common mistake is moving your knees inward. This can be detrimental to your knee joints. When you do a squat, push your knees outward with your kneecaps facing the same direction as your toes. Be careful not to extend your knees beyond your toes, as this may cause unnecessary strain and possible knee injury. While squatting, keep your back straight. Keep your head up, open your chest, and relax your shoulders. Do not bend or arch your back when you move into the squatting position. Finally, when you squat, make sure that your heels remain on the floor at all times. Do not lift up your heels, as this may lead to strains and injury and render the exercise ineffective.

Progressions

Chair Squats

If you struggle to do basic squats, chair squats are a good

option for practicing your form and execution. You will need a chair to perform this exercise.

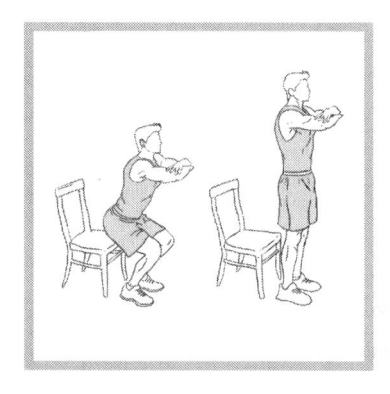

- Stand in front of the chair with your feet approximately shoulder-width apart and your toes pointing outwards.
- Proceed to do a squat. When you move down into a squatting position, stop before your glutes touch the chair.
- Proceed to raise your body into the starting position using your legs.

When you do the chair squat, imagine that you are going to sit on the chair. This mental visualization will help you to perform the exercise more effectively.

. . .

Variations

Once you can do at least ten squats with ease, there are several progressions that you can move on to. These progressions will improve your strength significantly.

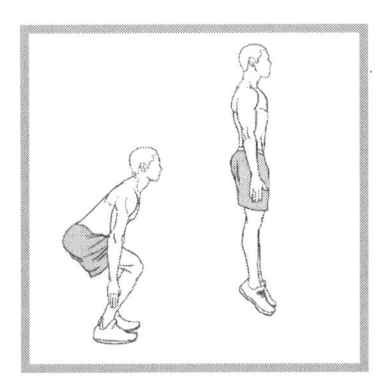

Jump Squats

Jump squats are similar to regular squats, but with an added jump at the end, this will improve your explosive power and build strength.

- Stand with your feet approximately shoulder-width apart, pointing your toes outwards.
- Bend your legs toward the floor and move into a sitting position. Keep your chest up and shift your weight to your heels.
- Pause with your knees over your toes.

- Using your legs, push yourself up with explosive strength into a jump. Jump as high as you can before proceeding to the starting position.

When you can complete ten repetitions of this exercise, you can then move on to the next progression.

Assisted Pistol Squats

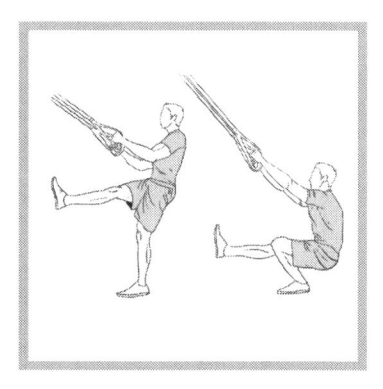

Assisted pistol squats will help you master the regular pistol squat more easily. These are executed with the same steps as regular pistol squats, with the exception that you hold on to something to stabilize yourself and maintain your balance. Refer to pistol squats for steps on how to proceed.

Once you can do ten assisted pistol squats effectively, you can proceed to attempt the pistol squat.

Pistol Squats

Pistol squats are quite tricky and can be arduous. Attempt this exercise with special care and mindfulness.

- Stand on one leg with your toes pointed forward.
- Extend one leg in front of you, keeping it as straight as possible.
- With all your weight on one foot, slowly sit into a squat. Keep your other leg extended and elevated.
- Use your grounded leg to push yourself up into the starting position.
- Alternate your legs and start again.

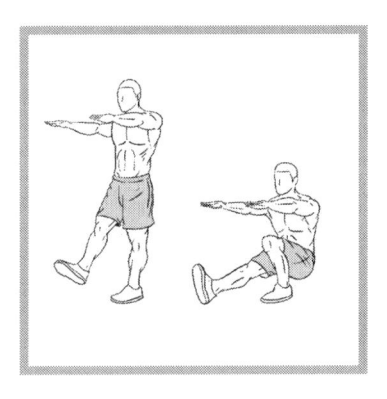

CORE EXERCISES

Lying Leg Raises

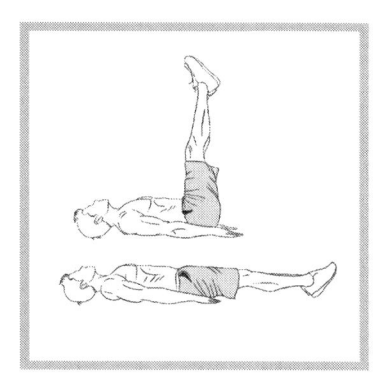

Core exercises focus mainly on building your core strength. That is, your back and stomach muscles. Leg raises are one of the main core exercises that can be done. There are countless variations of leg raises, but lying leg raises are the most basic. Lying leg raises are an excellent core-strengthening exercise and can be more complicated than they seem.

- Lay down with your back flat on the floor. Extend your legs and keep your feet together.
- Keeping your feet together and your legs straight, lift your feet in the air stopping at an angle of 30 to 45 degrees.
- Lower your legs down onto the floor without lifting or arching your back.

Doing this exercise wrong can cause severe spinal strain and can hurt your back. When doing this exercise, be careful to keep your lower back on the floor at all times. Do not arch your back during any point in this exercise, as this may cause injury. Keep your neck straight and do not lift your head. Remember to breathe during this exercise. Inhale when lowering your legs and exhale while raising them. Do not try to do this exercise too quickly. Move slowly and be mindful of your movements. This is how you will get the best results out of your leg raises.

Progressions

Regular leg raises can be very difficult for an amateur Calisthenic. If you find it difficult to do regular leg raises, try practicing assisted leg raises first.

Assisted Leg Raises

Assisted leg raises are similar to regular leg raises, but much easier. Assisted leg raises will help you master the basic movements of the leg raise without placing too much strain on your back.

- Find a surface such as a box, a bench, or a chair that will offer you something to lean your legs on.
- Lie with your back flat on the floor and elevate your legs against the box.
- Lift your legs to a 90-degree angle without arching your back. Keep your head on the floor.

- Next, lower your legs back toward the starting position. Do not let your legs fall. Focus your motion on your core, and try to maintain control of the exercise.

Once you are effectively able to do about ten assisted leg raises, doing lying leg raises should be easier.

Variations

Once you can do at least ten lying leg raises comfortably, you can then move on to more complex variations and will eventually be able to do hanging leg raises.

Parallel Knee Raises

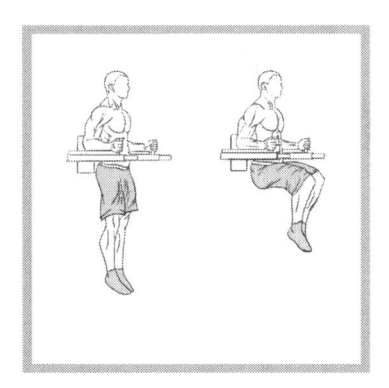

To do this exercise, you will need access to a dip bar, or some variation thereof. Parallel knee raises will help you develop your core and arm strength.

- Grasp the two parallel bars on either side of your body with your hands shoulder-width apart.
- Keep your arms extended, raise your feet off the ground, and bend your knees forward at a 90-degree angle.
- Raise your knees as close to your chest as possible.
- Keeping your knees bent, lower your legs slowly into the 90-degree position without letting your feet touch the ground.

Once you can do at least eight of these perfectly, you can move on to the next progression.

Parallel Leg Raises

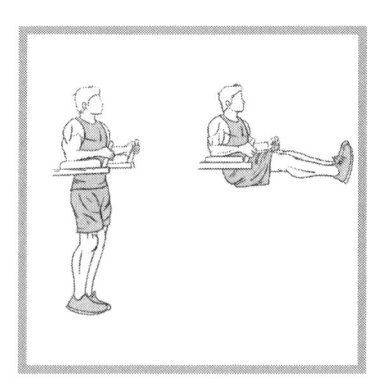

Parallel leg raises are similar to parallel knee raises, with the exception that your legs must be extended. This exercise increases the strain on your core and leg muscles.

- Grasp the two parallel bars on either side of your body with your hands shoulder-width apart.
- Keep your arms extended, raise your feet off the ground, and keep your legs extended.
- Raise your legs as far upward as possible without bending your knees.
- Lower your legs slowly without letting your feet touch the ground.

Practice this exercise until you can elevate your legs to a 90-degree position. When you can do eight of these exercises confidently, you can attempt the next progression.

Hanging Knee Raises

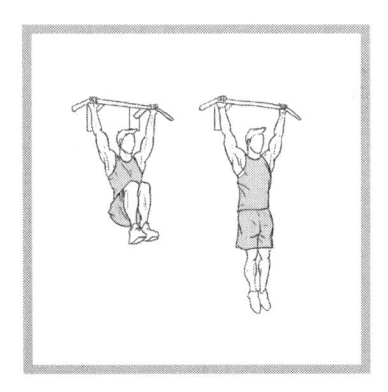

This exercise requires a pull-up bar. It is much more strenuous on the arm and core muscles as it is done from a hanging position. Hanging is hugely beneficial for your shoulders.

- Stand facing the vertical bar.
- Grasp the bar with your hands, keeping your arms slightly more than shoulder-width apart.
- Using your core strength, pull your knees up as close to your chest as possible.
- Lower your knees slowly into the starting position.

Once you can complete eight repetitions of this exercise, you can move on to the final progression.

Hanging Leg Raises

This exercise requires access to a pull-up bar. It is similar to the hanging knee raise, with the exception that the legs are fully extended.

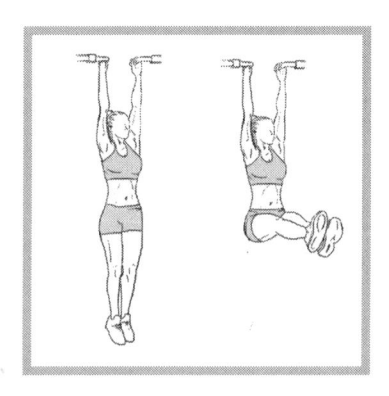

- Stand facing the vertical bar.
- Grasp the bar with your hands, keeping your arms slightly more than shoulder-width apart.
- Using your core strength, keep your legs as straight as possible and raise them as high as possible.
- Lower your legs slowly without bending them.

Ideally, you should be able to raise your legs to at least a 90-degree angle. From here, there are countless other complex variations and progressions that you can try.

Once you have successfully mastered the highest level of progression for each of these basic exercises, you are well on your way to becoming a master Calisthenic and fitness expert. Your goals are well within your reach.

3

GUIDANCE - THE ROUTINE THAT WILL GET RESULTS

So, you've just finished reading Chapter 2, and you're excited and motivated and ready to start. You realize, however, that you haven't actually done any exercise yet, and you don't know how to apply all the knowledge you've just learned. You may be asking yourself where to start, how many repetitions of each exercise to do, and how often to do them. You may be overwhelmed by all the possibilities and variations.

Developing your own workout routine can be difficult if you are not yet familiar with the basic movements of Calisthenics. This chapter will provide you with a basic routine, to begin with on your Calisthenic journey, as well as the equipment you will need to practice this routine. Once you have mastered these basic exercises, you can move on to try other exercises and variations and design your own workout routine. There are countless Calisthenic exercises, and these are but a few.

THE BASIC ROUTINE

This basic Calisthenic routine includes dips, pull-ups, push-ups, pistol squats, and hanging leg raises - all exercises you've just learned. These exercises have all been explained in the previous chapter. If you have just started your Calisthenics journey and are not yet familiar with designing your own workout routine, this routine will help you get the hang of the basic exercises and prepare for later progressions. Once you become familiar with these exercises, you can move up the progression scale and attempt more complex exercises and variations. The general rule of thumb is that if you can do ten repetitions of an exercise with ease, you can then move on to the next progression. If you are unable to do these correctly, however, try an easier progression first. This routine will increase your strength, endurance, and mobility. Pay particular attention to developing the correct form and technique for each of these exercises, even if it means doing only one or two repetitions of the exercise. Execution is more important than the number of repetitions you can manage.

The principle of this workout routine has been adapted from THENX recommendations (OFFICIALTHENX, 2017,

03:15–05:21). In this workout routine, you will work your way down the progressions of each exercise, starting with the most challenging progression you are capable of doing. Do as many repetitions of each progression as you can, then move down one progression until you reach the easiest progression of the exercise. Once you feel you've maxed out a particular progression, hold the extended position as long as possible before moving on. Do this until you have reached the lowest level of progression for the exercise, then take a 30-60 second break before you move on to the next exercise. If you have trouble moving between progressions, take a 30-second break between each exercise. You should aim for 3-5 cycles of this routine to feel the most benefit.

Dips

Start with the highest possible progression you can manage. If you cannot do a weighted dip yet, start with the highest possible level that you feel comfortable with doing. In time, you can focus on moving up the progression scale until you can do all variations of this exercise.

Start with weighted dips. Do as many of these as you can, hold the extended position, and then immediately move on to regular dips until you feel you can't do any more of these. Next, move on to negative dips and bench dips. Once you have successfully moved down the progression scale, take a 60-second break before moving on to the next exercise. It is not necessary to do assisted dips as part of your progression. Instead, these can be used to help you reach the level where you are able to do dips without the assistance of resistance bands.

Pull-Ups

Start this exercise with weighted pull-ups, do as many as you can, once you cannot do anymore hold the elevated position as long as you can, and then proceed to regular pull-ups. When you feel you cannot do any more of these, hold the elevated position, and then move down the scale to jumping pull-ups and eventually Australian pull-ups. Once you reach your limit, take a 60-second break before proceeding to the push exercises. You do not need to do assisted pull-ups as part of these progressions. Instead, use the exercise as a stepping stone to doing regular pull-ups. Once you can do regular pull-ups, you can ditch the resistance bands.

Push-Ups

Start this exercise with regular push-ups. Once you feel you've reached your limit and you've held the push-up position as long as you can manage, you can proceed to do high to low planks and, ultimately, knee push-ups. Incline push-ups are not necessary for this progression. These can be used to help you master the push-up. Once you have completed all these progressions to your maximum capacity, take a 60-second break.

Pistol Squats

For the next exercise, start with pistol squats, alternating your legs as you go. If you can't do regular pistol squats, you can substitute these with assisted pistol squats. Once you've maxed out on these and you've held the extended position as long as you can manage, you can move on to jump squats and then regular squats. Seated squats are meant to help you perfect your form when performing squats and need not be included in these progressions. Once you have worked your way down these progressions, rest for 60 seconds.

Hanging Leg Raises

The last exercise is hanging leg raises. Since the progressions discussed in Chapter 2 are so different from one another, this exercise will consist only of hanging leg raises and hanging knee raises. If you feel you want to add the parallel and lying leg raises, you are free to do so. Assisted leg raises are intended only to help you develop your form with lying leg raises and need not be added to the regimen. Once you have completed this section, complete 3-5 cycles, and then you have successfully completed your very first Calisthenic workout. Congratulations!

Remember to pay specific attention to form and execution.

Even if it means that you do the exercises slowly and can perform fewer repetitions, developing a solid form is fundamental to your development and progression. Holding the extended position before moving on helps the body build endurance, which will help when attempting more complex and taxing exercises.

OPTIMAL EQUIPMENT

You will need some equipment to complete this exercise routine. If you do not have access to the equipment or cannot afford to buy the equipment, however, there are some free alternatives that you can opt for that will be equally fitting.

For the pull-ups, dips, and leg-raise progressions, you will need a pull-up bar, a dip bar, and a lower parallel bar for Australian pull-ups, these could be in the form of the back of two chairs to perform dips or lower hanging clothes rail for Australian pull-ups. If you do not have access to these at home, you will likely find these in a park. You can easily use monkey bars for your pull-up exercises, and there should be some railings or lower bars for you to perform Australian pull-ups and two parallel bars for dips. Some places have even erected playground-themed exercise parks. These parks have make-shift gym equipment that uses bodyweight instead of adding weights to the equipment. These parks are environmentally friendly and usually open to the public, and they can be a good alternative if you don't have access to the necessary equipment. You will also need a weighted belt to perform weighted dips and pull-ups. If you do not have access to a weighted belt, you can use a weighted vest or even a loaded backpack to add weight to your exercises. The possibilities are endless, and there are countless alternatives to consider when doing Calisthenics training. The main advice here is to be creative; there is always furniture around your home; you can turn into make-shift gym equipment, and if not, a park is a safe bet for the equipment you will need.

With this exercise routine and the equipment to help you, you should be well on your way to becoming a regular Calisthenic. Once you have mastered these exercises, you can start at higher variations like the diamond push-up and L-sit dips. You can then move on to develop your very own exercise routine and attempt more complex Calisthenic exercises and variations.

4

DEVELOPMENT - CONTROLLING YOUR OWN PROGRESSION

Once you have mastered the basic movements and are comfortable with these movements, you can then move on to constructing your own training routine. Constructing your routine doesn't just happen, however. Several things must be considered when you plan your routine. Take careful note of these before you construct your training routine. Keep in mind that your routine should be adapted or altered once you start to feel too comfortable with the movements. The aim is to encourage progression and improvement, not to make exercise easier. My hope is that by showing you that these exercises are, in fact, possible, you will realize that with the right kind of Mindset, you will be able to reach your goal.

BUILDING YOUR OWN EXERCISE ROUTINE

When constructing your own exercise routine, there are several things that you should keep in mind and consider. These factors will have a direct impact on the way that your exercise routine is structured. Before we start, it is important to note that training consists of a number of cycles. Macro-cycles are long-term periods of three, six, or twelve months. These are directly linked to your long-term goals. Your macro-cycles should be flexible, however, as your routine will inevitably be adapted according to your progression and development. Micro-cycles, on the other hand, are the workouts that are to be completed every week. Both of these cycles are important to keep in mind when you plan your workout routine, as your micro-cycles will directly affect the outcome of your macro-cycle in the long run.

SETTING GOALS

Setting a goal is the first crucial step in constructing your exercise routine. It is extremely important to know what you are working toward before you plan your new exercise routine. Whatever goal you are aiming toward will ultimately determine the type, level, and intensity of your exercises. Without a goal, you will have no specific direction, no measure of progress, and nothing to remind you why you are doing this in the first place. It is also much easier to become demotivated, as progress can sometimes be slow and not as clearly visible. Goals are an excellent way to keep us on track and motivate us to keep on going when we feel like giving up. Here are some examples of how goal setting will influence your workout routine:

1. Strength:

Strength training requires a low number of repetitions paired with a high number of sets. Typically, strength training requires doing your repetitions with as much weight as possible, or in the highest possible progression. Rest periods are significantly longer in strength training since exercises are much more taxing on your muscles.

2. Endurance:

Endurance training requires a combination of strength and cardio workouts. High-Intensity interval training (HIIT) is a good example of this kind of exercise. These exercises would require a reduced rest period and can include explosive exercises such as explosive pull-ups. Compound movements are a good option for endurance training. Finally, it is important to alternate and change exercises to prevent your body from getting too used to any particular workout or exercise.

3. Weight loss:

Weight loss training is similar to endurance training, with less focus on strength. Training for weight loss would require high-intensity exercises that hike up your heart rate. Short rest periods force your body to recover much quicker. Whole-body exercises are best for weight loss, as they target all the muscles and areas of your body. Another good strategy that you may apply is doing cardio exercises such as jogging on your rest days.

4. Achieving specific movements:

Training to achieve certain movements such as the muscle-up can require a split-body approach that focuses on specific movements and muscle groups at a time. Split-body training versus full-body training is discussed in more detail in Chapter 6.

That being said, deciding on a long-term, far-off goal is not enough. Long-term goals can be a good yardstick in the long run, but setting smaller, short-term goals will keep you motivated, help you celebrate your milestones, and help you measure your progress more easily. It is, therefore, important to set both long-term and short-term goals.

Long-term goals should drive your macro-cycle - your long-term aim like building strength - and will determine the kind of exercises you plan for your exercise routine. Short-term goals should be revised and set weekly to help you keep track of your progress and keep you motivated. Completing 5 push-ups with perfect form by Friday would be a good short-term goal. Having a better picture of your short-term progress will significantly improve your determination and help you to stay focused on the bigger picture - the long-term goal.

There are some principles or strategies that you may wish to keep in mind when setting your goals.

Firstly, it is important to be specific, especially in your short-term goals. If your goals are not specific enough, they might be hard to attain or measure, which will inevitably demotivate you in the long run. Your goals should be something measurable and easy to define. Rather than stating that you want to exercise more regularly, for example, make your goal specific and measurable by saying that you want to exercise at least three days a week. This is something you can easily measure and cross off.

Secondly, make sure that your short-term goals line up with your long-term goals. Short-term goals should be a stepping stone to help you achieve your long-term goals and should keep you motivated enough to get there.

Your goals should be challenging. The purpose of setting goals is to help you improve and develop. Therefore your goals should challenge you to go beyond your current ability and do more and better than you are currently doing. Your goals should not be unattainable, however, which leads us to the next principle.

Be realistic! Unrealistic goals will leave you more demotivated than ever as they might not be achievable. Your goals should be an encouragement rather than a stumbling block.

Very importantly, you should write down your goals somewhere where you can see them on a daily basis. This will help motivate you to reach your goals. Keeping track of your goals, even the ones you have managed to achieve, is an effective way to keep yourself motivated and excited. It will also make you more aware of your actions, challenging you to do better daily.

Goal-setting is an integral part of your exercise regimen as it determines the type, frequency, and volume of your workout routine. It will also help you to stay motivated and excited, encouraging you to do better. With the right goals, you will soon be on the right track to achieving your desired physique and fitness level.

Weaknesses

Identifying your weaknesses is not only an exercise strategy; it is a commonly applied principle. Identifying gaps can help you to improve in weaker areas and complete exercises more efficiently.

Imagine a hypothetical construction worker named Bob, who was bad at laying foundations, but he could pack a brick wall like nobody's business. So instead of working on improving his foundation-laying skills, Bob decided to stick to what he does best. So, he lays the foundation the same way every time or just ditches the foundation altogether. Instead, Bob focuses on what Bob does best - packing brick walls. Ignoring the foundation isn't going to prevent the building from caving in.

In the same way, ignoring your weaknesses will get you nowhere. You need to be working on these areas until they're no longer an area of concern. Determine what is keeping you from achieving your goal and making the progress that you feel you should be making, and then strategize on how to overcome the issue. If you have trouble finding these areas of weakness by yourself, you might want to do more research, ask a friend, or consult a specialist to help you identify them.

Frequency

It is important to be realistic about the frequency of your workouts. If you know that you are a busybody and a workaholic, select a frequency that is realistic and fits into your schedule. You can always work in an extra session or two, rather than having to skip sessions that were planned. If you do have time to exercise every day of the week, however, remember that rest is an essential factor in muscle recovery and muscle building. I have touched on the physiology behind muscle building in Chapter 1 and will elaborate on the importance of rest in Chapter 8. If you insist on training every day, make sure that your workouts consist of various levels of intensity. Try alternating intense full-body workouts with less intense skill sessions where you try to master difficult moves rather than working your body hard, or try breaking your workouts into push, pull, legs to give each muscle group at least 48 hours rest. Intense exercise every day of the week will not only burn you out rapidly, but you will soon experience a plateau in your rate of progression. This is because your body's rate of muscle damage is higher than the rate of repair, leaving your body in a destructive state.

Rest

Rest periods between repetitions should be as short as possible. Shorter rest periods often produce better results and increase endurance, although they can be slightly longer for strength training. Take between 30 and 60 seconds of rest between repetitions to produce optimal results. Shorter rest periods force the body and muscles to adapt and speed up the recovery rate. Furthermore, you should plan to have rest days in between your sessions as well. I have alluded to the importance of rest in recovery, and taking a day off, or at least including a low-intensity workout, is a very important part of the recovery process.

Intensity and Volume

Intensity considers the extent of the strain that an exercise places on your body. More intense exercises might involve adding extra weight or doing a complex progression of the exercise. Volume, on the other hand, concerns the number of repetitions that you perform in a set. When you plan your intensity and volume, it is essential to note that both of these factors cannot be high at the same time. It is highly unrealistic to plan your workout with both high intensity and high volume simultaneously. High intensity is likely to focus more on developing strength, whereas high volume will likely increase your fitness and endurance levels, burning fat and getting you shredded.

Another important thing about volume is that, whatever amount of repetitions you decide to do, you should be able to perform them with perfect form. Planning a set with a high volume of repetitions is unrealistic if you are unable to execute the exercise with the correct form. You may be able to do the repetitions, but using an incorrect or inconsistent form will limit the outcome of the exercise and can easily lead to strains, pains, and injury.

Tempo

The tempo of an exercise entails how quickly it is done. It is important to note that a higher tempo does not automatically equal better results. On the contrary, performing exercises at a slower tempo with a focus on form is likely to produce better results than exercises performed with a focus on speed executed with inconsistent form. A higher tempo often helps to increase fitness and endurance levels. High-tempo exercises should only be adopted once the correct form has been mastered.

Each micro-cycle should focus on three main factors - range of motion, skill, and strength. These three factors work together to ensure the optimal outcome for each exercise. It is important when you do an exercise that you complete the full range of motion for each exercise. Failing to do so will reduce the benefits of the exercise and limit your progress significantly. Completing your exercises with the full range of motion will increase your muscle flexibility and can reduce the risk of injury. Furthermore, a full range of motion makes exercises more intense and therefore maximizes the benefits.

Performing exercises with skill and precision takes time, dedication, and a lot of practice. Performing an exercise with the correct form and skill is invaluable, however, and will allow you to maximize your results. Strength is developed by using the right approach and the right kind of exercise. By applying THENX's workout strategy, as discussed in the previous chapter, you will condition your body to reach the optimal strength level. Therefore, when you design and plan your micro-cycles, pay specific attention to range of motion, skill, and strength, and how these factors will be used to achieve the maximum benefits from the workout.

5

EVOLUTION - ACHIEVING NEXT-LEVEL MOVEMENTS

BUILDING TOWARD MORE INTENSIVE EXERCISES

If you have purchased this book, the chances are that you've seen videos on YouTube of Calisthenic athletes doing ridiculously insane and remarkable moves. You probably looked into Calisthenics because you want to master the same kind of impressive moves. This section will provide you with some examples of how to use progressions to learn more complicated exercises. These examples will not only help you master these exercises yourself, but will also give you some ideas of how to structure your routine to achieve your goals.

The Front Lever

The front lever is an exercise that requires you to hold yourself in a horizontal position, seemingly only using your arm muscles, but a strong core will be the key to its success. This is one of the most advanced Calisthenic exercises. Since the front lever works against the force of gravity, this exercise becomes increasingly difficult the taller and heavier you are. Don't worry if it seems like it's taking a long time to master, morethanlifting.com suggests that learning to do the front lever can take a good six months ("How To Front Lever: The Complete Beginner's Guide," n.d.). If your core, back, and arm muscles are strong enough, you can use the following steps to work your way up to the front lever. Practice each step until you feel comfortable moving on to the next one. If you cannot yet do step one of these progressions, refer to Chapter 2 for some easier progressions. Once you can do hanging raises, you will be well on your way to achieving the front lever.

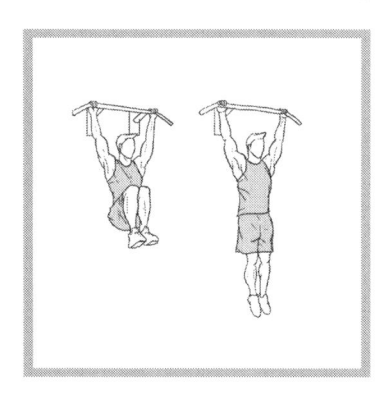

Step 1: Hanging Knee Raises

These will help you to strengthen your core muscles. You will need access to a pull-up bar.

- Stand facing the vertical bar.
- Grasp the bar with your hands, keeping your arms slightly more than shoulder-width apart.
- Using your core strength, pull your knees up as close to your chest as possible.
- Once you have reached the elevated position, lower your knees slowly into the starting position.

You should be able to do at least eight hanging leg raises with perfect form before proceeding to the next progression.

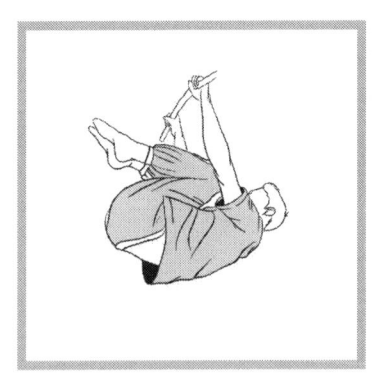

Step 2: Tuck Front Lever Hold

This exercise will significantly develop your arm, back, and shoulder strength. You will need to strengthen these muscles considerably to perform the front lever. You will need a pull-up bar to complete this exercise.

- Stand facing the bar and grasp the bar with your hands slightly more than shoulder-width apart.
- Tuck your knees into the elevated knee raise position.
- Using your arms and core, and keeping your arms extended, slowly raise your body into a horizontal position with your back as parallel with the floor as possible. Keep your knees in a tucked position.
- Once your back is parallel to the floor, hold this for as long as you can

Your arms should remain straight, and your knees tucked throughout the exercise. Once you can comfortably hold this for 20 seconds, you should be able to proceed to the next progression.

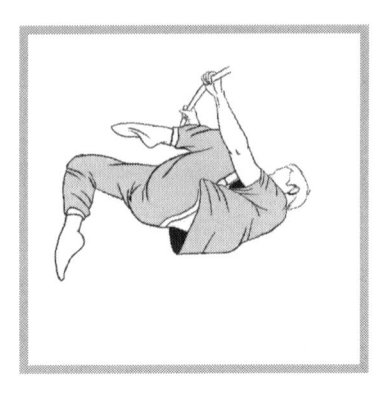

Step 3: Tuck one leg Front Lever

This exercise will focus on developing your ability to hold yourself in the lever position.

- Stand facing the bar and grasp the bar with your hands slightly more than shoulder-width apart.
- Tuck your knees into the elevated knee raise position.
- Using your arms and core, and keeping your arms extended, slowly raise your body into a horizontal position with your back as parallel with the floor as possible. Extend one leg bent from the tucked position.
- Hold this position for as long as you can manage, keeping your back parallel to the floor.

Once you can hold this position for 10 to 15 seconds, you may proceed to the next progression.

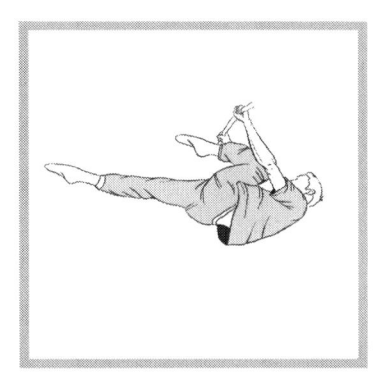

Step 4: Alternating Front Lever

This progression will help you get used to the extended leg movement and strengthen your core enough to support your body weight in the front lever position.

- Stand facing the bar and grasp the bar with your hands slightly more than shoulder-width apart.
- Tuck your knees into the elevated knee raise position.
- Using your arms and core, and keeping your arms extended, slowly raise your body into a horizontal position with your back as parallel with the floor as possible.

- Holding this position, extend one leg while keeping the other retracted.
- Alternate your legs, keeping your body parallel to the floor.

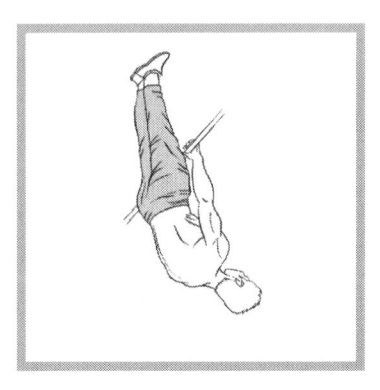

You may find it easier to perform the negative by extending your legs vertically in the air above your head and the pull-up bar, then try slowly lowering your leg extended position down into the horizontal position.

Once you can complete this exercise with ease for at least 10 seconds, keeping your body parallel to the floor, you may proceed to the next and final progression.

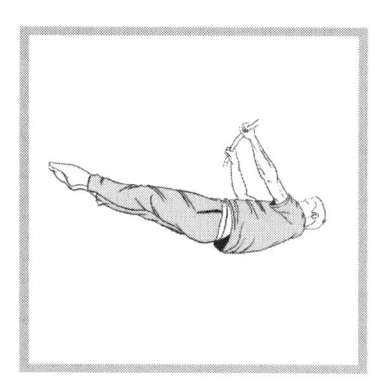

Step 5: The Front Lever

- Proceed to the elevated front lever hold.
- Spread both your feet as you extend your legs while holding the parallel position. Doing this will help to disperse the tension throughout your body, rather than focusing the tension on your core.
- Once you can manage this, bring your legs closer together until they are completely together.

Once you can bring your legs together, you have achieved the front lever.

The Human Flag

The human flag is what it sounds like. The exercise is performed by placing both hands on a vertical pole and lifting (and holding) your body parallel to the ground in a flag-like fashion. This exercise requires tremendous core strength and works on all the major body muscles. When you attempt this exercise, you will probably do better to position your dominant arm at the top rather than the bottom to ease your grip and hold. Al Kavadlo (2017) suggests five progressions to help you master the human flag. You will need a vertical bar to complete all of these progressions.

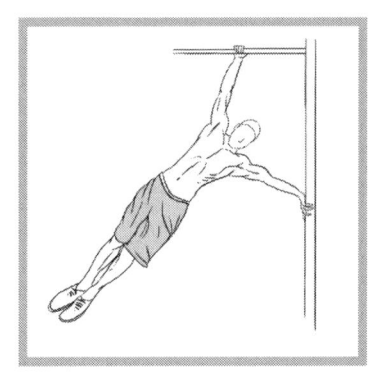

Step 1: The Support Press

This progression will require access to a pull-up bar with vertical support.

- Grab the horizontal pull-up bar with one hand and use your other hand to press into the vertical support bar.
- Keep both of your arms extended and keep your

shoulders and lats engaged.

- Keeping both your feet together, lift your feet off the ground as you press into the vertical bar while pulling from the horizontal pull-up bar.
- Tense your body without bending your elbows, and keep yourself at a 45-degree angle to the ground. Hold this position.

Once you can hold this position for at least 20 seconds, you should be able to move on to the next progression.

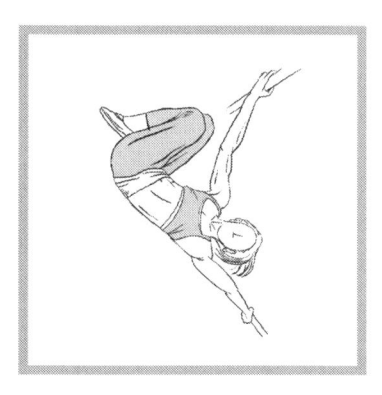

Step 2: The Chamber Hold

This step will require a pull-up bar with vertical support and an additional horizontal bar much closer to the ground.

- Grasp the top vertical pole with one hand, and the

lower vertical pole with the other hand positioned directly under the top hand.

- Jump up and kick your legs to lift your hips in the air, slightly higher than shoulder-height.
- Press into the bottom pole with your bottom arm and simultaneously pull with your other arm. Keep your knees tucked in close to your body.
- Hold this position, keeping both your arms fully extended throughout the exercise.

You should be able to hold this position for at least 10 seconds before attempting to move on to the next progression.

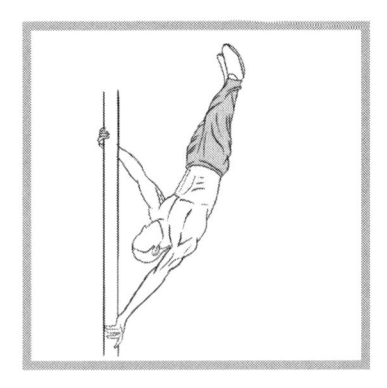

Step 3: The Vertical Human Flag

The vertical human flag is similar to the chamber hold, but

your legs should be extended. This exercise aims to keep your body as vertical as possible.

- From the chamber hold position, slowly extend your legs upward and hold the position.
- Aim to start as vertical as possible, moving toward a more diagonal angle as you progress.

Once you can hold the vertical human flag position for at least 10 seconds, you can proceed to the next progression.

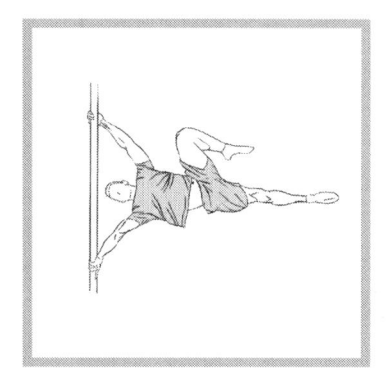

Step 4: Bent Knee Flag

From the vertical human flag position, lower your hips down to a horizontal position with one or both legs tucked in. You can start this exercise with both legs tucked and then move on to alternating your leg tuck, keeping one leg extended while the other is in a tucked position.

Once you can hold this position comfortably, you can then move on to the next and final progression.

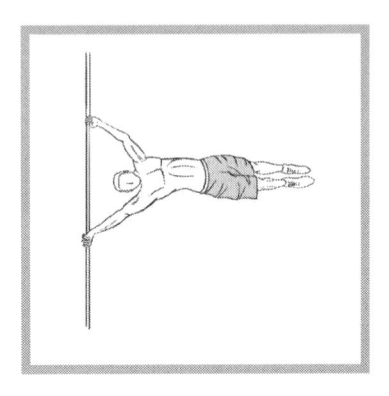

Step 5: Human Flag

The human flag position can be approached in one of two ways: a top-down or bottom-up approach. The bottom-up approach is significantly more complicated than the top-down. Therefore, start with the top-down approach to help you gain control over your body and ease your body into the exercise. Once you have mastered the top-down approach effectively, you may then proceed to attempt the bottom-up approach.

Top-Down:

The top-down approach is designed to increase the load on your body gradually. Starting from a vertical human flag position, gradually lower yourself into the human flag position. These movements should be slow and deliberate to maintain control of your body and ease yourself into position.

Bottom-Up:

This method involves starting from the floor and pushing yourself up into the horizontal human flag position. Having to start from a neutral position makes this approach significantly harder, but also more impressive and effective.

For both of these approaches, you should push into the pole as much as possible using your bottom arm and pull using your top arm. This will keep you elevated and stable, enabling you to hold the position. Keep your whole body tense during the exercise to achieve full control and maximum core activation. One thing to keep in mind is that the closer your torso and legs are to the pole, the more leverage you will have.

The Muscle-Up

Muscle-ups can be done using a pull-up bar or gymnastics rings. Since the use of gymnastics rings is significantly more complicated, however, this section will focus on using a pull-up bar to execute this exercise. Doing the exercise on bars first will ease the process of learning to do it on rings. Dr. Allen Conrad (Lindberg, 2019) suggests practicing the following exercises to help you prepare for the muscle-up:

Step 1: Swinging Knee Raises

This exercise is similar to a hanging knee raise, but with an added twist motion to help strengthen your core. You will need a pull-up bar to complete the exercise.

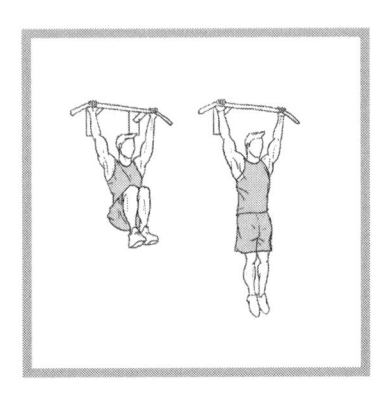

1. Stand facing the vertical bar.
2. Grasp the bar with your hands, keeping your arms slightly more than shoulder-width apart.
3. Using your core strength, keep your legs as straight as possible and raise them as high as possible, twisting your sides as you raise your legs.
4. Lower your legs slowly without bending them.

Once you can do eight of these with ease, you can move on to the next level.

Step 2: Pull-Ups

This exercise will help to improve your core and arm strength.

- Stand facing the pull-up bar.
- Grasp the bar with your hands, keeping your arms slightly more than shoulder-width apart.
- Pull yourself up using your shoulder muscles, raising your head above the bar.
- Then, lower yourself slowly using your arms and core.

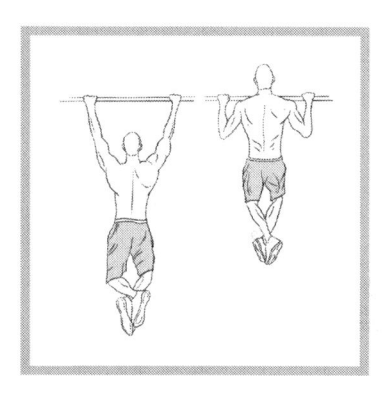

These should be executed perfectly, using the correct form and method. You should be able to do at least ten-twelve pull-ups using the proper form and execution before attempting the muscle-up.

Step 3: Tricep Dips

This exercise can be done using dip bars or with two chairs on either side of you.

- Grasp the two parallel bars (or chairs) on either side of your body with your hands shoulder-width apart.
- Raise your feet off the ground with only your arms to support your weight. Keep your knees slightly bent backward and legs crossed. Keep your elbows slightly bent at all times.
- Lower yourself by bending your elbows until your arms are at a 90-degree angle.
- Now, use your arms to push yourself up toward the starting position.

Practice doing at least ten-twelve tricep dips using the correct form and method.

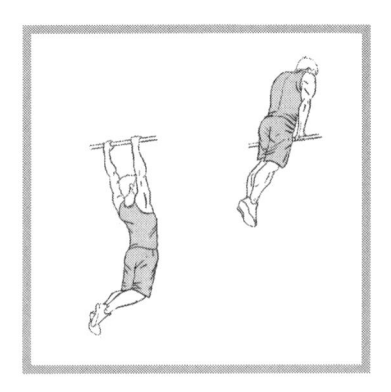

Step 4: The Muscle-Up

Once you have executed these three exercises effectively, comfortably, and with perfect form, you should be prepared to attempt the muscle-up. To perform the muscle-up, follow the steps outlined below:

- Hold the pull-up bar with your thumbs on top of the bar rather than around it.
- Pull yourself up to a pull-up position.
- Twist your wrists and position your chest over the pull-up bar.
- Perform a tricep dip and lower yourself back into the hanging pull-up position.

By mastering pull-ups and tricep dips, you should have the skills capable of doing a muscle-up, then by continuing to perform muscle-ups, you will be able to increase your repetitions. But going straight to the muscle-up may be too difficult, if that is the case, attach a resistance band and practice doing the muscle-up with this assistance, slowly reduce the resistance band level till you can perform a muscle-up naturally with no assistance.

The Iron Cross

The iron cross is typically done using gymnastics rings. This exercise places tremendous pressure on your joints, so you need to be sure that you are, in fact, ready to attempt this exercise. Pull-ups and muscle-ups are good exercises to prepare you for the iron cross. If you cannot execute these with perfect form yet, do not attempt the iron cross. However, if you can then, as suggested by Maurice (2019), here are the 7 steps to help you achieve the iron cross.

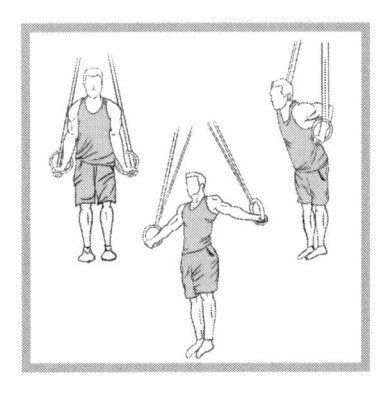

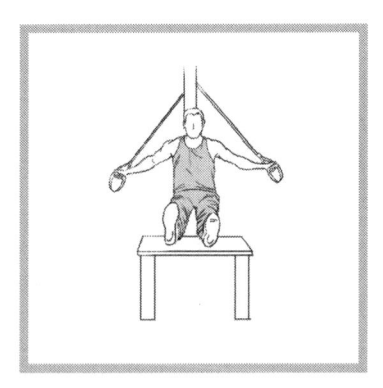

1. Start by hanging on the gymnastics rings with the rings about waist height, arms fully extended, and

elbows locked out. Hold this position as steadily as possible for about 5 to 10 seconds. Once you can manage to hold this position for 20-30 seconds with stable hands, try swinging your body slightly while maintaining stability. When you've managed to effectively swing your body whilst maintaining your balance and stability, proceed to step two.

2. Practice doing dips on the rings while maintaining your stability. If you can't manage to do dips on the rings, practice doing them on the bars first. If you can do ten-twelve dips on the bars, you should be ready to attempt them on the rings. Once you can do eight-ten dips on the rings with ease, you can move on to the next progression.

3. Place a table or support block around waist height in front of you. Hold on to the rings and elevate your feet onto the table or block. Move your body down into the cross position and push yourself back up. As you progress, move the table or block backward until only your toes are leaning on the block.

4. Using the same block progression, do the exercise with only one leg extended at a time. Alternate your legs to ensure that both legs are evenly strengthened.

5. Now, practice moving your body down into the

cross position and back up without the additional support.

6. Once you can do this effectively, repeat the exercise and hold the cross position for at least 5 seconds before you dropdown.
7. You should now be able to do the iron cross completely.

The Superman Push-Up

Before you can do the Superman push-up, you need to be able to do basic push-ups with ease and precision.

Practice clapping push-ups before you attempt to do the Superman push-up. These will help you get used to pushing your upper body off the ground.

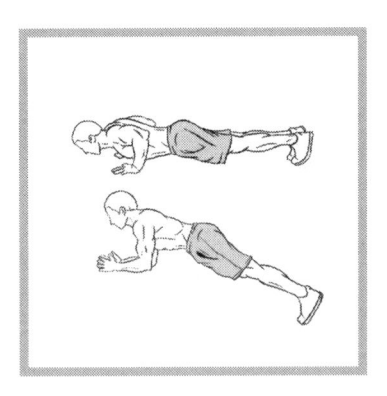

The clapping push up:

- Start in the regular push-up position, with your legs extended and your arms stretched out in front of you.
- Bend your elbows and lower yourself toward the floor until your chest almost touches the floor. Keep your core tight throughout the movement.
- Push your body upward with explosive force using your hands and propel your upper body into the air.
- Keep your feet on the floor and clap your hands together before landing back in the starting position.

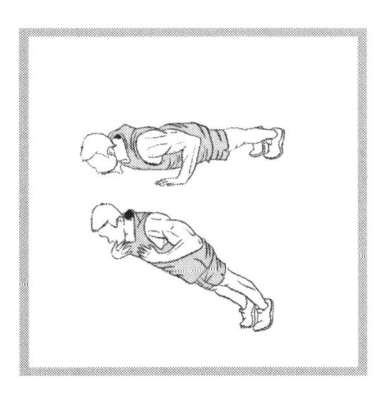

The chest tap push up:

- Start in the regular push up position.

- Bend your elbows keeping them tucking into your torso till your chest is almost touching the floor
- Then push upwards with explosive force and aim to touch your chest with both hands before returning to the ground and push up position.

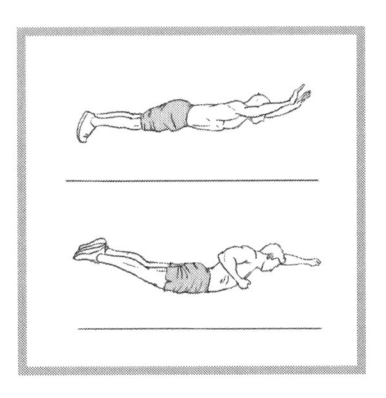

The Superman push up :

Once you have mastered these progressions, attempting the Superman push-up should be significantly easier. It may be hard to bring yourself to leave the ground with both your arms and legs as nobody wants to end up with a face full of floor, so try leaving the ground without extending your arms first then follow the following instructions for the superman push-up:

- Start in the regular push-up position, with your

legs extended and your arms stretched out in front of you.
- Bend your elbows and lower yourself toward the floor until your chest almost touches the floor. Keep your core tight throughout the movement.
- Push your body upward with explosive force using your hands and feet, propelling yourself into the air.
- Once your hands and feet lift off the floor, extend your arms and legs into a flying position with your body extended in a straight line.
- Land back in the starting position as you hit the ground and start your next repetition.

The 90-Degree Push-Up

The 90-degree push-up is an extremely taxing exercise that requires an immense amount of strength, balance, and control. It combines the handstand, push-up, and planche exercises to form an impressive and extremely difficult full-body exercise. There are a number of progressions that you can practice to help you execute the 90-degree push-up.

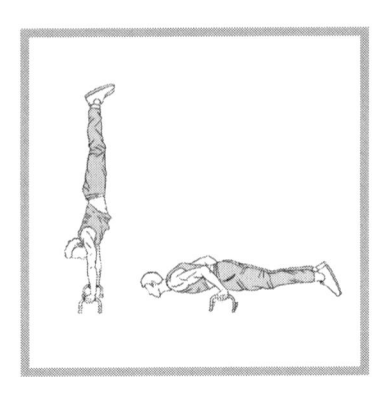

The push-up and 90-degree hold:

- Starting in the push-up position, lower your body into a push-up.
- Next, lean your body forward, shift your weight onto your arms, and lift your feet off the floor. Keep your body parallel to the floor.
- Keep your arms bent and hold that position as long as you can.
- Release the position and repeat.

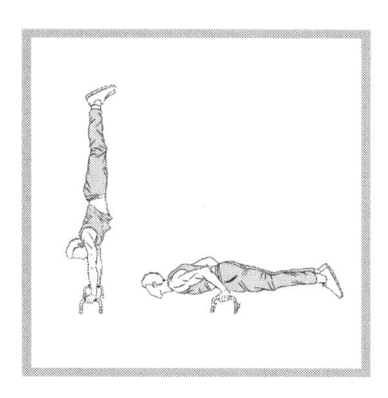

The negative 90-degree hold:

- Using your legs, kick your body into the handstand position.
- Lower your body into the Planche position using your arms and core strength, and hold this position as long as you can.
- When you can't hold this position any longer, release your hold and start again.

The negative 90-degree hold isolates the part of the exercise where you need to lower yourself into the Planche position and focuses on developing the strength to execute that part of the exercise. In doing so, you reduce the number of techniques you need to develop and focus on when you finally attempt the 90-degree push-up.

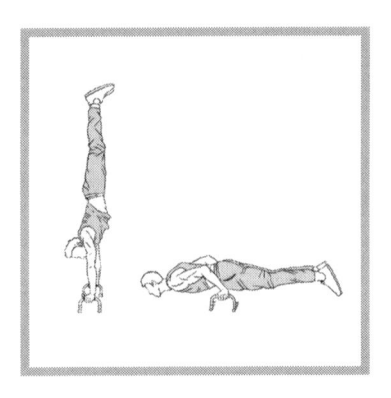

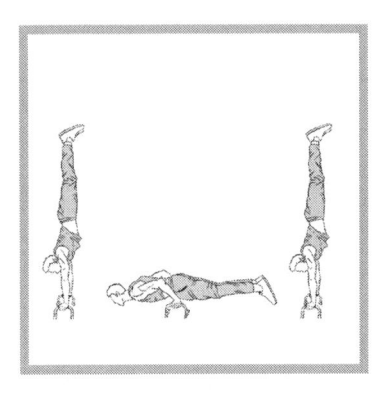

The 90-degree press:

- Position your body in the starting push-up position.
- Lean forward and shift your body's full weight onto your arms.
- Raise your legs off the ground and proceed into the handstand position.
- Next, lower your body into the Planche position

using your arms and core strength and hold this position as long as you can.
- When you can't hold the Planche position any longer, release your hold and start again.

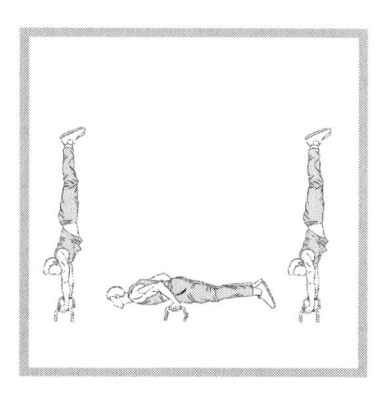

The 90-degree push-up:

- Starting in the push-up position, elevate your body into a handstand position. Keep your entire body in a straight line.
- Next, use your arms to lower yourself as you would in a handstand push-up and lower your body into the planche position.
- Once you've reached the full planche position with your body at a 90-degree angle to the floor, use your arms and your legs to push yourself back into the handstand position.

- Once you've reached the handstand position again, repeat steps two and three. Other than your hands, your body should not touch the floor during any part of this exercise.

The Planche

The planche is an insanely intense exercise that will help you develop tremendous arm, wrist, and shoulder strength. Mastering the planche is no easy feat and will take a significant amount of patience and determination. Several progressions will help you work toward mastering the planche. Some of the basic exercises that you need to master before you attempt the planche are the plank, push-up, pull-up, and dips. If you are comfortable with each of these exercises and can execute them using perfect form, there are five progressions that you can practice to prepare you for the planche.

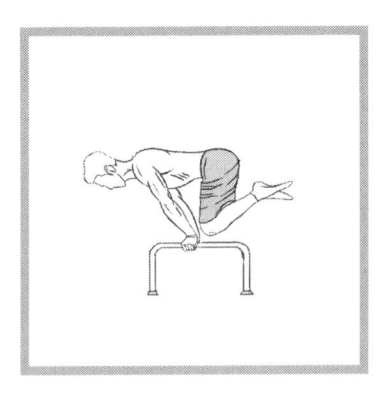

Step 1: The Frog Stand

- Take up the full squat position and place your hands on the ground in front of your feet. Support your elbows by resting them against your knees.
- Lean forward and place your body's full weight onto your hands.
- Lift your feet entirely off the ground and hold this position. Your shins should be parallel to the floor.

You should be able to hold this position for at least 60 seconds before moving on to the next progression.

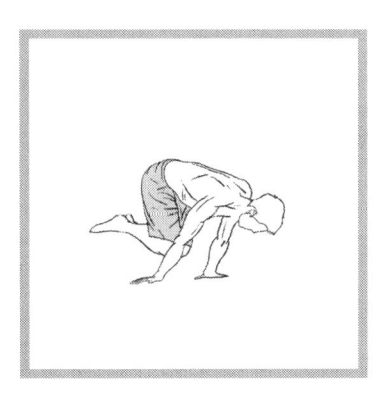

Step 2: Tuck Planche

The tuck planche is similar to the frog stand, with the exception that your knees should be tucked into your chest so that your extended arms are entirely supporting your body weight.

- Take up the full squat position and place your hands on the ground in front of your feet.
- Lean forward and place your body's full weight onto your hands.
- Lift your feet entirely off the ground. Curve your back and tuck your knees into your chest. Hold this position for as long as possible.

Once you can hold the tuck planche for at least 60 seconds, you may then proceed to the next progression.

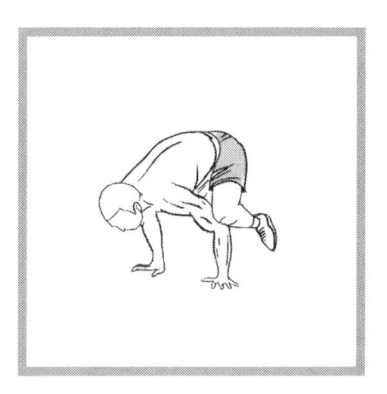

Step 3: Advanced Tuck Planche

The advanced tuck planche differs from the tuck planche,

mainly in the positioning of the back. Whereas the tuck planche is performed with a curved back, the advanced tuck planche requires that you straighten your back.

- Start by executing a tuck planche.
- When you have reached the tuck planche position, extend your hips above and behind you until your back is straight. Hold the position for as long as possible.

Once you can hold the advanced tuck planche for 60 seconds, you should be able to move on to the next progression.

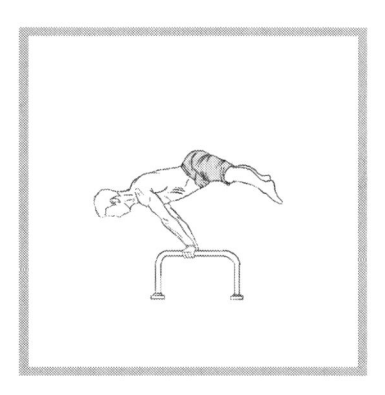

Step 4: Straddle Planche

- Move into the tuck planche position.

- From this position, slowly extend your legs from your chest straight behind you. Spread your legs as you extend them.
- As you progress, attempt to bring your legs closer together. You will need to lean forward to maintain your balance and compensate for the shift in weight.

If you can hold the straddle planche for at least 10 seconds, you can proceed to the next and final progression.

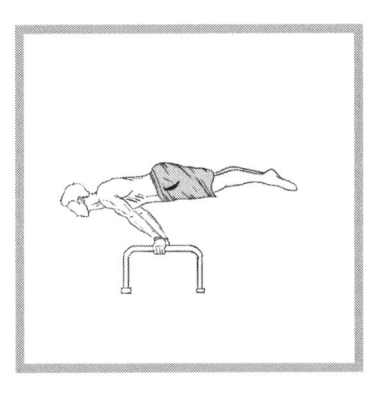

Step 5: The Planche

The full planche is almost similar to the straddle planche. The only difference is that your legs should be held together while you hold your position.

- Place your hands on the floor in the push-up position.
- Lean forward, shifting your entire body weight onto your arms.

Keeping your legs together, raise your whole body off the floor, keeping it as parallel to the floor as you can. Hold this position for as long as possible.

6

EVALUATION - TARGETING YOUR WEAKNESSES

You may need to strengthen specific areas or muscles to be able to complete a certain movement or exercise, such as the ones mentioned in Chapter 5. In this case, you may need to adopt a split approach in your exercise routine. If you are not sure whether you should adopt a split- or full-body approach, consider the pros and cons of each.

SPLIT VS. FULL-BODY WORKOUTS

Both full-body and split-body training can be beneficial. One is not necessarily better than the other. These approaches will depend on the kind of goals you are aiming to achieve. There are several differences, pros, and cons to each of these training strategies.

Split-Body Training

Split workouts are best for strengthening certain areas or muscle groups in your body. They are a good strategy to help you progress within skills or movements, such as the muscle-up or the planche. Split workouts help you to work on your weaknesses and help you achieve certain movements. Split workouts focus on training different muscle groups or movement patterns in each workout session. Most commonly, workouts are split by either muscle groups or movement patterns such as push or pull exercises.

Split workouts are often used by fitness models, bodybuilders, or advanced lifters who want to focus on developing certain muscles or movements at a time. These kinds of workouts can also be beneficial for those of you who want to build strength or muscle beyond the level that full-body workouts provide. This is not to say full-body workouts cannot build strength and muscle, but you can provide more attention to each muscle group with split workouts by performing more exercises that train that muscle group.

The benefits of split workouts are that they can be done in greater volume while still providing plenty of rest for each muscle group, which can promote more muscle growth. Split workouts are versatile and easy to change up, so your body is less likely to get used to the exercises, and you are less likely to get bored with your exercise routine. Split workouts offer more time for your central nervous system to recover since it focuses on different muscle groups. You are, therefore, also far less likely to overtrain. Split-body training is good for body-shaping, focusing on specific areas of your body. Lastly, because it focuses on different muscle groups at a time, split-body training is not as taxing and easier to manage.

Some cons must also be considered, however. Split-body workouts burn fewer calories and therefore does not burn body fat as effectively, so it will be harder to shred down. Split-body training can quickly cause muscle or strength imbalances if certain muscle groups are trained more than others. Since split-body training focuses on different muscle groups in every workout, you cannot easily skip workouts. It will mean that certain muscle groups are being neglected as you do not work that muscle group as frequently as with full-body training.

So split training can be beneficial for intermediate level trainers and above as you should have already built up a well-proportioned body. You can then use split training to target muscle groups you want to improve for your aesthetic or to develop an advanced movement.

Full-Body Training

Full-body training focuses on training the whole body in

every workout. It develops full-body strength and promotes overall progression.

Cardio fanatics often uses Full-body workouts as they are metabolically intensive. This kind of workout strategy is recommended for beginner or intermediate trainees.

A full-body workout strategy is very convenient for those who keep busy schedules, as it does not require as frequent exercises as split-body workouts. Depending on the intensity of your workouts, full-body workouts can be done between three and five times per week. It is therefore not necessary to train every day. Full-body training promotes higher levels of energy expenditure, which promotes rapid fat burn and better hormonal balance. Full-body training is beneficial to your overall health as it develops the entire body. Full-body training is also more likely to offer you a balanced body, both aesthetically and on a muscular level.

Full-body training does not allow you to focus on certain muscle groups and is, therefore, not as efficient in developing certain muscle groups or movements. Furthermore, due to the intensity of full-body training, it can easily lead to overtraining if you do not allow your body enough rest.

These two approaches are therefore used for different reasons, and both can be effective depending on your goals. For weight loss and an all-round improvement in strength and physique, full-body training would be the best option. It is also recommended for beginners and intermediate trainees, but the military uses full-body training, so advanced trainers should not feel as though it is not for them too. If you are looking into achieving certain movements or improving specific muscle groups, however, split-body training would be the better option. Beware of focusing too much on one particular group of muscles, however, as doing so will leave you imbalanced and may lead to muscle weakness in other areas. A huge part of Calisthenics is trying to maintain the most proportioned body as this is the most healthy and aesthetically pleasing, so whatever training you do, make sure you maintain this balance.

Split-Body Workout Routines

Split-body workouts can be tricky if you've never done them before. It can be challenging to determine which workouts will best develop which areas or movements. This section will provide you with some examples of workouts that focus on push and pull movements, and core and leg muscles. Ensure that you warm up before each of these workouts to prevent unnecessary injury and improve results. These exercises can be adapted or changed to suit your specific needs, but they are a good starting point for anyone who is unsure of which exercises to do to develop certain movements.

PULL WORKOUT

Pull workouts focus on developing your pull-movements, such as pull-ups. I will provide you with a workout routine suggested by Saturno Movement (2018, 03:15–05:21) that will help you to improve your pulling strength significantly. This exercise can be completed in sets according to the specifications in each exercise or circuits.

Exercising in sets involves completing a set amount of repetitions a certain amount of times before moving on to the next exercise. You will, therefore, complete the total number of sets for one exercise before moving on to the next exercise. If you choose to complete this exercise in sets, rest for 30-60 seconds between sets and 1-2 minutes between exercises.

Circuit workouts involve completing one set of each exercise until you have completed all the exercises, and then starting again. The workout is thus repeated in its entirety for a certain number of sets.

Repetitions and sets can be adapted according to your needs or ability. Choose the progression that best suits your ability level.

Explosive Australian pull-up

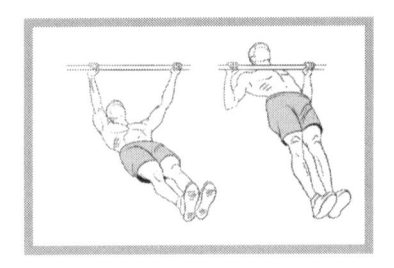

This exercise should be done until you feel fatigued or lose your explosive strength since the focus is on explosive movements. Four to six repetitions are recommended in five sets, but this can be adapted according to your needs. You will need a vertical bar at about chest height to complete this exercise.

- Stand facing the pole and grab the pole with both hands, arms extended.
- Lower your body at an angle that is comfortable for you, with your legs extended and dig your heels into the ground. The higher the angle, the easier this exercise will be.
- Using your arms, pull your chest as explosively as possible toward the bar and slowly lower yourself back to the starting position.

If this exercise is too easy for you, you might try to do explosive pull-ups. You will need a pull-up bar to complete this exercise.

- Stand facing the pull-up bar and grab the bar with both hands.
- Grasp the bar with your hands, keeping your arms slightly more than shoulder-width apart.
- Using your arm, back, and shoulder muscles, pull your body up as high and explosively as possible.
- Lower yourself slowly using your arms and core.

Explosive pull-ups can also be done in five sets with four to six repetitions.

Negative Tuck Front Lever

This exercise will require two parallel vertical bars at the same height as the one used in the body rows; dip bars will work. Four to six repetitions in five sets is the recommended volume of the exercise, but this can be adapted as needed.

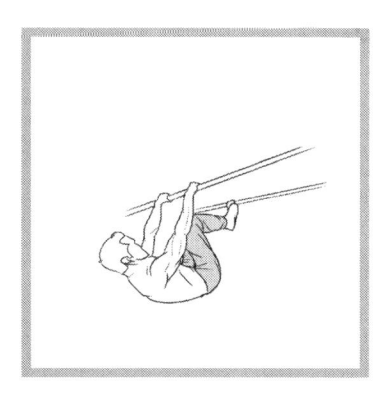

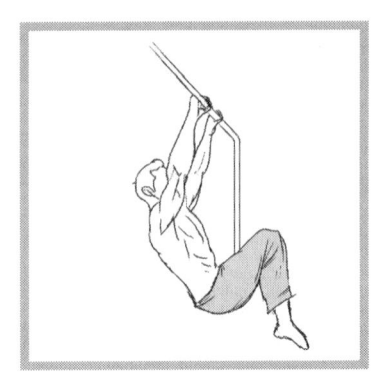

- Stand facing the bar and grip the bar with both hands, arms extended.
- Place your feet on the opposite bar, bending your knees at a 90-degree angle. Your back should now be parallel to the floor.
- Supporting your body with your arm and back muscles, bring your knees in close to your chest. At this point, only your arms should be holding onto the bar.
- Lower yourself slowly until your feet reach the floor.

A more advanced progression of this exercise is tuck front lever raises. These can be done using a pull-up bar.

- Stand facing the bar and grip the bar with both hands, arms extended.

- Pull your knees up into a 90-degree position.
- Using your arms and core, slowly raise your body into a horizontal position until your back is parallel with the floor. Keep your knees in a tucked position.
- Once your back is parallel with the floor, slowly lower your body back into the vertical position.
- Keep your arms straight and your knees tucked at all times during the exercise.

Do this exercise with four to six repetitions in five sets.

Wide/Close Grip Negative Pull-Ups

You will need a pull-up bar to complete this exercise. The recommended volume for this exercise is eight repetitions in three sets for both the wide and close grip pull-ups. This exercise is the same as a jumping pull up, but with your arms positioned at a wide and close grip, respectively.

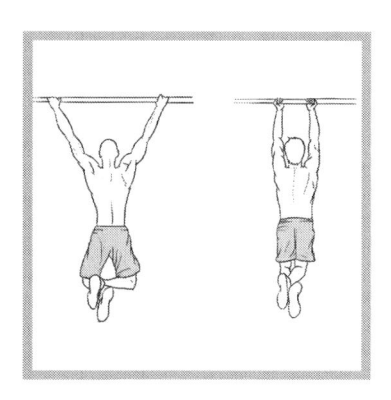

- Stand facing the vertical bar.
- Grasp the bar with your hands at a wide grip.
- Jump up into the elevated pull-up position.
- Lower yourself slowly using your arms and core, and let go once you have completely lowered your body.

Once you have done the eight repetitions, complete the exercise again with a close grip.

A more advanced version of this exercise would be wide/close grip pull-ups. You will need a pull-up bar for this exercise.

- Stand facing the pull-up bar.
- Grasp the bar with your hands with a wide grip.
- Pull yourself up using your shoulder muscles, raising your head above the bar.
- Then lower yourself slowly using your arms and core.

Once you have completed the eight repetitions, repeat the exercise with a close grip. This exercise may be completed with eight repetitions in three sets for each of the grips.

Reverse Flyes

THE GYM-LESS WORKOUT

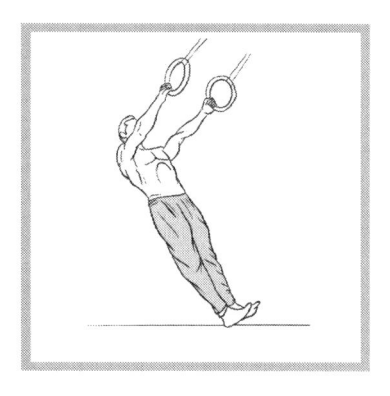

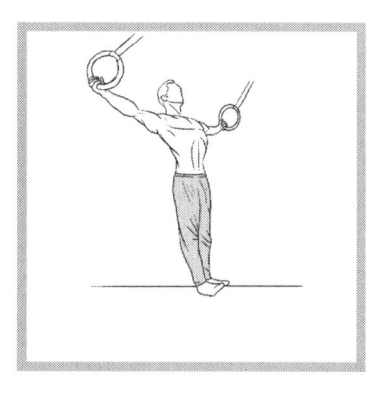

To do this exercise, you will need access to gymnastics rings. It is recommended to do this exercise with ten repetitions in three sets.

- Stand facing the rings and grab hold of the rings with your arms extended.
- Lean back while digging your heels into the floor, keeping your body straight. Adjust the angle of your body to make the exercise easier or more

difficult. The higher the angle of your body, the easier the exercise will be.
- Pull yourself up using your arms and core until your arms are extended horizontally in a cross position.
- Move slowly back into the starting position.

You should maintain total control throughout this exercise.

This exercise can alternatively be done in an upright position using resistance bands or equipment cables. If you are using resistance bands, stand on the resistance bands and pull the bands back using opposite hands. Equipment cables should also be crossed over for optimal resistance. You can also put two bedsheets or big towels over a door and close the door leaving you with the longer sides hanging down the door, hold the ends and step back until they are taut, then follow the steps above.

For an easier alternative, or if you do not have access to any of the equipment above, you can also do dumbbell reverse flyes with either dumbbells or water bottles.

- Sit on the edge of a bench or chair. Your dumbbells or water bottles should be placed on the floor behind your heels.

- Lean as far forward as you can, keeping your back straight and pick up the dumbbells or water bottles.
- Bending your elbows slightly, lift the dumbbells as far as you can, squeezing your shoulder blades together and slowly lower your arms again. Keep your back straight as you do this exercise.

This exercise can also be done in a standing position.

- Hold the dumbbells or water bottles in either hand with your arms extended in front of you.
- Pull your arms backward, squeezing your shoulder blades, until your arms are at a 180-degree angle.
- Slowly bring your arms back into the starting position and repeat.

Whichever alternative you opt for, complete ten repetitions in three sets.

Body Rows

To do this exercise, you will need gymnastics rings or bedsheets, as mentioned before. Do eight repetitions of this exercise in three sets.

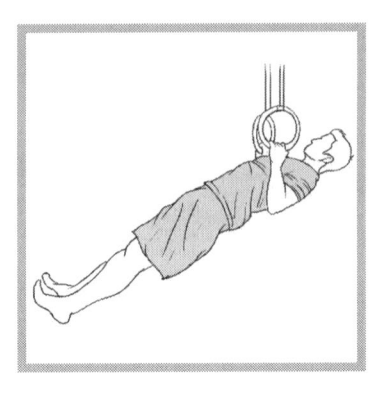

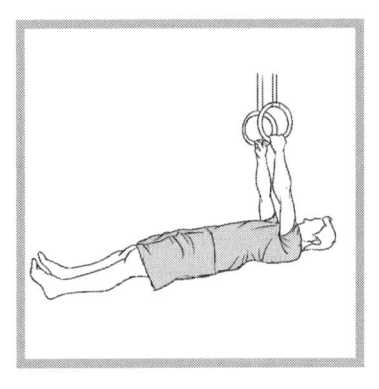

- Hold on to the rings with both arms extended and lean back with your heels digging into the ground. The angle of your body will determine the difficulty of the exercise. A lower angle would be more difficult.
- Keeping your body straight, use your arms to pull your body closer to the bar, starting from a pronated grip (overhand grip) and moving to a neutral grip (same way you would grip a ski pole) as

you pull up. Bend your elbows and squeeze your shoulder blades as you pull yourself closer.
- Slowly lower yourself back into the starting position.

For a more advanced alternative, you can do single arm body rows. This exercise can be done using gymnastics rings or a vertical bar. Using gymnastics rings would be significantly more difficult.

- Holding on to the ring or bar, with your arm extended, lean back with your heels digging into the floor. Again, your angle will determine the difficulty of the exercise.
- Keep your legs about shoulder-width apart to maintain your balance.
- Keeping your body straight, starting with a pronated grip as you use your arm to pull your body closer, changing to a neutral grip. Bend your elbow and squeeze your shoulder blade.
- Slowly lower yourself back into the starting position using your arm.

Do this exercise with eight repetitions for each arm in three sets.

Negative Chin-Up

This exercise is done with a specific focus on the pull and release movements involved in executing the chin-up. This exercise can be done in intervals of 5-to-10 seconds, depending on your ability, and only one set. You will need a pull-up bar for this exercise.

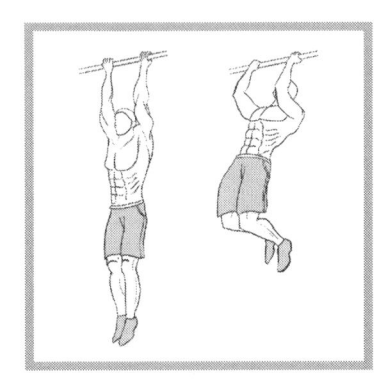

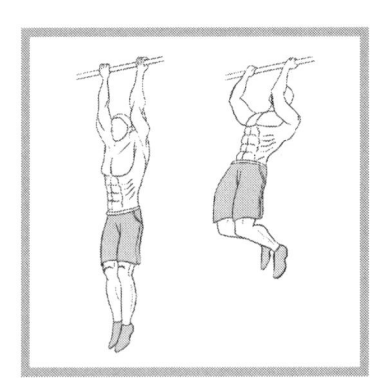

- Stand facing the vertical bar.
- Grasp the bar with your palms facing toward you. Keep your arms slightly more than shoulder-width

apart.
- Jump into the elevated chin-up position and hold this position for 5 to 8 seconds.
- Slowly, for a period of 5 to 8 seconds, lower yourself back into the starting position.

A more advanced alternative to this exercise is the slow chin-up. This exercise can be done in periods of 10 seconds, or 20 seconds for more advanced trainees. You will need a pull-up bar for this exercise as well.

- Stand facing the bar and hold the bar with palms facing toward you, arms slightly more than shoulder-width apart.
- Slowly, for a period of either 10 or 20 seconds, raise yourself using your arms and core strength until your chin is above the bar.
- Hold this position for 10 or 20 seconds.
- Slowly, for a period of 10 or 20 seconds, lower yourself back into the starting position.

This exercise requires only one set, as the focus is on developing strength and endurance in the movements involved in the execution of the exercise.

Ring Curls

This exercise requires access to gymnastics rings or similar alternatives, as mentioned reverse flyes. To make the exercise easier, you can adjust the angle of your body. A higher angle would be easier, while lowering the angle of your body makes the exercise harder. This exercise can be done with ten repetitions in four sets.

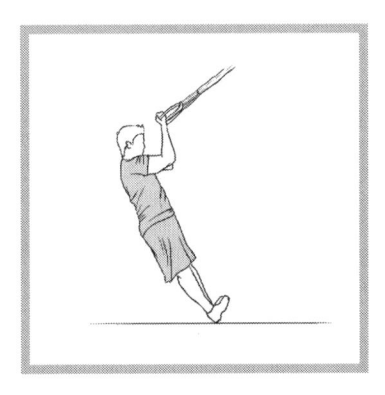

- Stand facing the rings. Grasp the rings or bed sheets with a supinated grip (underhand grip) with your arms extended and your elbows pointing toward the floor.
- Lean back with your heels digging into the floor. Adjust the angle according to your difficulty level.
- Keeping your biceps at a 90-degree angle with your body, curl your arms to bring the ring to your forehead.
- Slowly move back into the starting position,

keeping your biceps at a 90-degree angle throughout the exercise.

For a more advanced alternative, you can do a single-arm ring curl.

- Stand facing the ring. Grab the ring with one arm extended and your elbow pointing toward the floor.
- Lean back with your heels into the floor. Keep your legs about shoulder-width apart to maintain your balance. Again, the angle can be adjusted according to the desired difficulty level.
- Keeping your bicep at a 90-degree angle with your body, curl your arm to bring the ring closer to your forehead.
- Slowly move back into the starting position, keeping your bicep at a 90-degree angle.

Do ten repetitions for each arm in four sets.

This workout can either be done in sets or in-circuit form, depending on your exercise goals and needs. You can reduce or increase the number of circuits or sets depending on how challenging you are finding it. If some of the moves are too difficult for you, then go back and continue using the full-body workout, as mentioned in Chapter 3, and master those progressions before coming back to this workout.

PUSH WORKOUT

This workout is another workout recommended by Saturno Movement (2018b, 03:15–05:21). These exercises focus mostly on developing push-movements such as push-ups. This exercise can also be completed either in sets or in-circuit form, depending on your goals or preferences. Little or no rest is recommended in between exercises, with two to three minutes rest between each circuit. However, this can be adjusted depending on your goals.

Repetitions and sets can be adapted according to your needs or ability level. Choose the progression that best suits your ability level.

Clapping Push-Ups

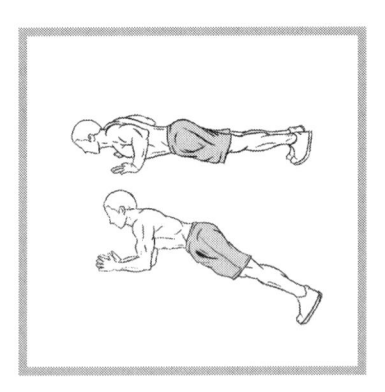

This exercise focuses on developing your explosive strength. Do six repetitions of this workout in five sets.

- Position yourself on the floor on all fours. Place your hands slightly more than shoulder-width apart.
- Extend your legs backward in such a way that you are balanced on your hands and your toes. Keep your body straight - don't raise or lower your back.
- Bend your elbows and lower yourself toward the floor using your arms until your chest almost touches the floor.
- Push yourself up as fast and explosively as you can, releasing your hands off the floor and clap your palms together.
- Land with your hands back on the floor in the starting position.

If this exercise is too easy for you, you might attempt explosive straight bar dips. This workout requires one dip bar.

- Face the bar and grip the bar with both hands.
- Push yourself off the floor, extending your arms and tucking your elbows inward.
- Using your arms, slowly lower yourself, leaning

your upper body forward to maintain your balance. Keep your back and legs straight at all times.
- Once you have lowered yourself as far as you can manage, push yourself up as fast as you can without losing control.
- Repeat the exercise

A more advanced version of this exercise will include releasing the bar when you push yourself up. Do this exercise with five sets of six repetitions.

Negative Tuck Planche Raise

To execute this exercise, you will need two parallel dip bars. This exercise can be completed with eight repetitions in three sets.

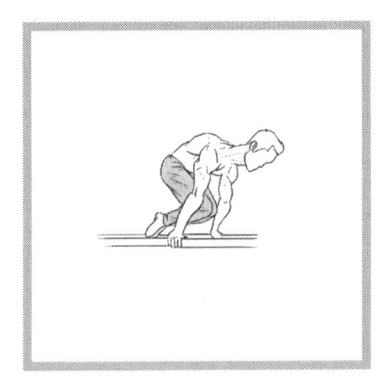

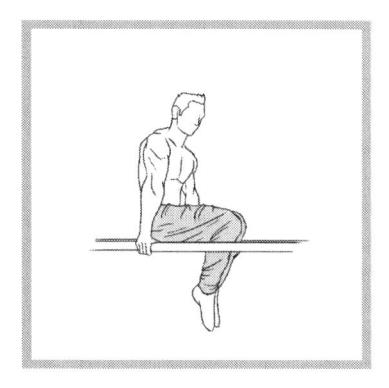

- Place your hands and your feet on the respective dip bars.
- Slowly tuck your feet into your chest, keeping your arms extended, so you are in the horizontal tuck position.
- Using your arms, slowly lower yourself to the floor.

A more advanced version of this exercise is the tuck planche raise, which is essentially the opposite of what I just described. This exercise also requires access to a dip bar.

- Place your hands on the dip bars, extend your arms so your legs are dangling in the air, and you are in the vertical position.
- Tuck your legs into your chest and hunch your back slightly.
- Push your body parallel to the floor by pushing

with your arms and leaning forward. Once you are parallel to the floor, lower yourself back into the vertical position.

If this exercise is still too simple, you may attempt advanced tuck planche raises, straddle planche raises, or full planche raises.

Do this exercise with eight repetitions in three sets.

Pike Push-Up

This exercise can be done in three sets of eight repetitions and requires no equipment.

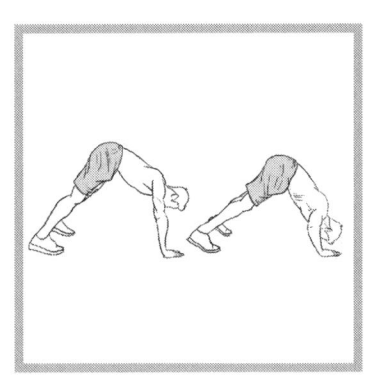

- Start in the downward dog yoga position, bending at the waist, until your hands are on the floor approximately shoulder-width apart.
- Keeping your back and your legs straight, lean

forward and bend your elbows to bring your crown as close to the floor as you can manage.
- Using your arms, push yourself back to the starting position.

You can also do these in an elevated position to make them more challenging. Place your legs on an elevated surface like the arm of a sofa, with your hands on the floor.

A more advanced alternative to this exercise is the handstand push up.

- Start in the standing position. Place your hands on the floor and kick yourself into a handstand.
- Keep your spine and legs straight, and your toes pointed. Use your arms to lower your head as close to the floor as possible.
- Use your arms, shoulders, and core to push yourself back up into the handstand position.

Do eight repetitions of this exercise in three sets.

Ring Chest Fly

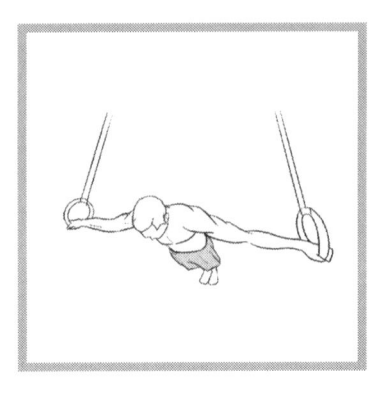

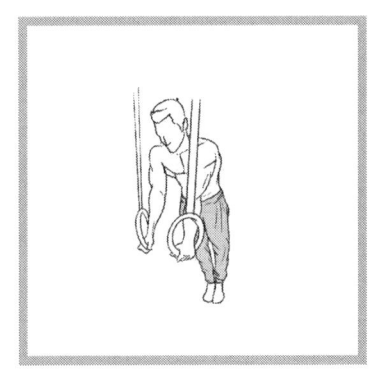

This exercise requires access to gymnastics rings sitting at about hip height. Alternatively, use the bed sheet method. Do this exercise with eight repetitions in three sets.

- Stand facing the rings. Grip the rings with your arms extended and your legs straight. Lean into the rings.
- Lean forward and slowly move your arms into a

horizontal position until your arms are at a 180-degree angle.

- Use your arms to push yourself back into the starting position, until your arms are straight. You should keep your arms straight and maintain control throughout the movement.

If you do not have access to gymnastics rings, this exercise can also be done in an upright position using dumbbells or water bottles.

- Stand up straight with your arms extended forward, holding the dumbbells or water bottles.
- Keeping your arms straight, slowly move your arms into a horizontal position, squeezing your shoulder blades, until your arms are at a 180-degree angle.
- Slowly bring your arms back into the starting position, keeping them straight and elevated at all times.

Push-Up

This exercise requires no equipment. It should be done with six repetitions in sets of three.

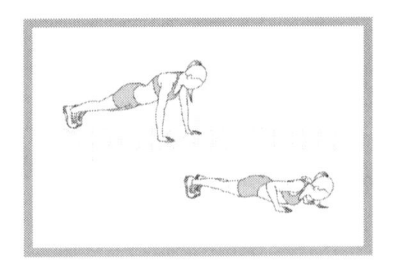

- Position yourself on the floor on all fours. Position your hands slightly more than shoulder-width apart.
- Extend your legs backward in such a way that you are balanced on your hands and your toes. Keep your body straight - don't raise or lower your back.
- Bend your elbows and lower yourself toward the floor using your arms until your chest almost touches the floor.
- Raise yourself again by pressing up with your arms until you reach your starting position. Your back should remain straight throughout the entire exercise.

An easier alternative would be to do knee push-ups.

- Position yourself on the floor on all fours. Position your hands slightly more than shoulder-width apart.
- Cross your legs in the air with your knees on the

floor. You should be balanced on your hands and knees only. Keep your back straight during the exercise.

- Lean your body forward, bend your elbows, and lower yourself toward the floor using your arms until your chest almost touches the floor.
- Raise yourself again by pressing up with your arms until you reach your starting position. Your back should remain straight throughout the entire exercise.

A more advanced alternative to the push-up is one-arm push-ups, but you could try diamond push-ups, clapping push-ups, or decline push-ups too.

Whichever alternative you choose, you should complete six repetitions in three sets.

Slow Dip

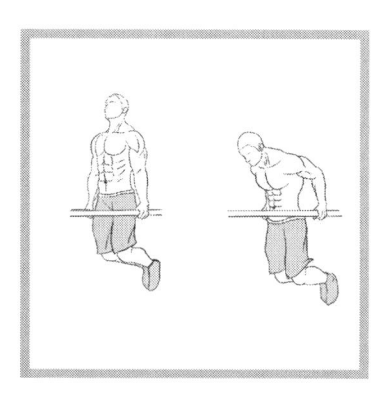

This exercise focuses on the movements of the dip exercise, developing strength and muscle endurance. Only one repetition is necessary in intervals of 30 seconds. You will need a dip bar for this exercise.

- Grip the bars on either side of you and extend your arms so that your legs are dangling.
- Using your arms, lower yourself slowly for a period of 30 seconds as far down as possible without touching the floor.
- Hold the lowered position for 30 seconds.
- Slowly raise yourself toward the starting position for a period of 30 seconds.

An easier alternative of this exercise is to do the exercise in intervals of 10 seconds for beginners, or 20 seconds for intermediate trainees. Only one repetition is necessary.

Skull Crusher

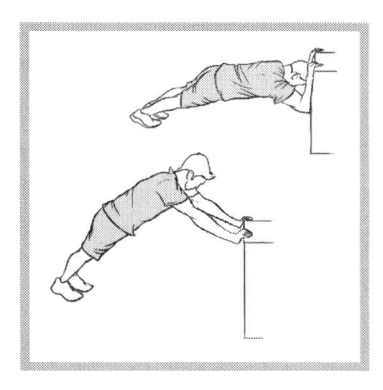

You will need a vertical bar or raised surface for this exercise. For a beginner-level exercise, use a higher bar or surface. A lower bar is more difficult. Do this exercise with ten repetitions in four sets.

- Hold on to the bar with arms extended. If necessary, you might have to position yourself on your toes, depending on how low the bar is.
- Keeping your body straight, bend your arms, and lean forward to bring your head to the bar.
- Use your arms to push yourself back up.

As with the pull workout, this set of exercises can be done in either circuit-style or sets. The number of repetitions and sets can be adjusted according to your needs and goals.

CORE WORKOUT

Core workouts focus on developing your stomach and back muscles. This exercise was recommended by Chris Heria (CHRIS HERIA VLOGS, 2019, 03:15–05:21) and is suitable for all levels of trainees. This workout requires no equipment and can be done anywhere.

Do this workout in a circuit style, doing all the exercises first and then repeating all of them again. Repeat the circuit four times.

Leg Raises

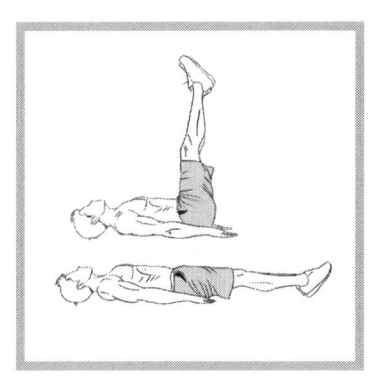

Do twenty repetitions of this exercise.

- Lay down on the floor with your back raised

slightly. Extend your legs and keep your feet together.
- Keeping your feet together and your legs straight, lift your feet in the air stopping at an angle of 30 - 45 degrees.
- Lower your legs down onto the floor without arching your back.
- Repeat the exercise.

This exercise can also be done on a platform to ease the execution of the exercise. Once completed, move on to the next exercise.

Leg Flutters

twenty repetitions are the recommended volume for this exercise.

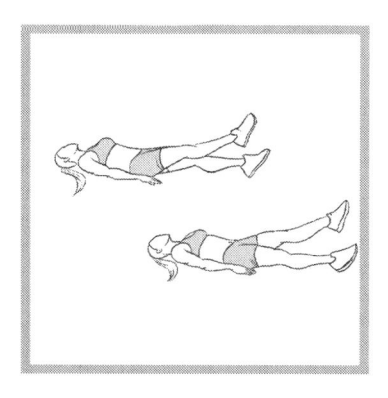

- Lay down on the floor with your back raised slightly. Extend your legs.
- Lift your right leg as far as you can, and hover the left leg just above the floor.
- Sitch your legs, lowering your right leg to a few inches above the floor and raising your left leg as high as possible. Keep both of your legs straight throughout this exercise.

Do this exercise on a platform to make the execution easier. Once you have completed twenty repetitions, move on to the next exercise.

Boat Hold

This exercise should be held for 25 seconds.

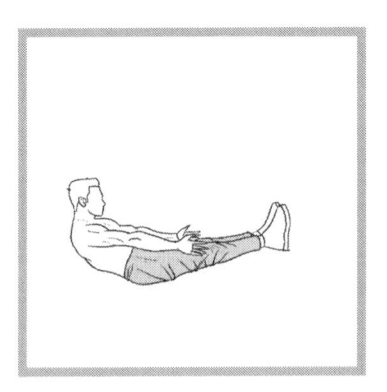

- Sit on the floor with your knees bent and your feet on the floor.
- Lean back slightly. Extend and raise your legs slightly.
- Extend your arms to maintain your balance and hold this position for 25 seconds. Keep your back and legs straight.

This exercise can also be done on a platform. Once you have held the position for 25 seconds, move on to the next one.

Russian Twists

This exercise can be done in thirty repetitions, fifteen repetitions on each side.

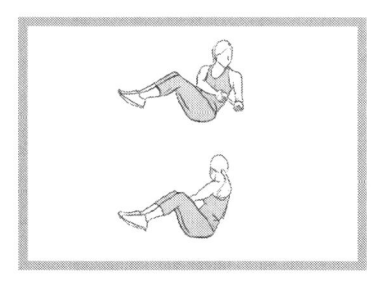

- Sit on the floor with your knees bent and your feet flat on the floor.
- Keeping your spine straight, lean back slightly, creating a v-shape between your thighs and torso.

- Bend your elbows and bring your hands close together.
- Twist your upper body from side to side, touching the floor with your hands as you reach each side. Keep your back leaned backward and your spine straight throughout the exercise.

To make this exercise more challenging, raise your feet so that only your heels are on the ground. Once completed, proceed to the next exercise.

Plank Side-to-Side

This exercise should be done in forty repetitions with twenty repetitions on each side.

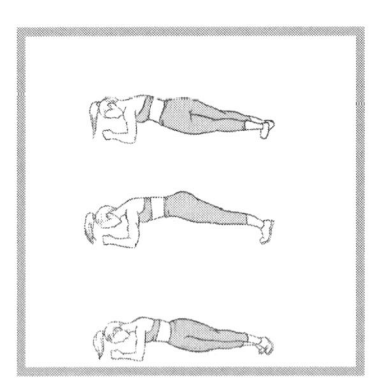

- Position yourself on your elbows with your legs extended. Keep your body straight.

- Dip your hips on one side toward the ground without raising or lowering your back. Twist your legs and abdominals as you dip your hips.
- Move back to the starting position and dip your hips toward the other side toward the ground.
- Repeat this exercise for the specified number of repetitions.

Once you have completed the exercise, move on to the next one.

Plank Side Hold

Hold this exercise for 30 seconds on each side.

- Position yourself on your side with your forearm flat on the floor and your elbow directly under your shoulder. Extend both legs with your feet stacked on top of each other.
- Lift your hips off the floor so that your body is straight.
- Hold this position for 30 seconds.
- Switch to the other side and repeat.

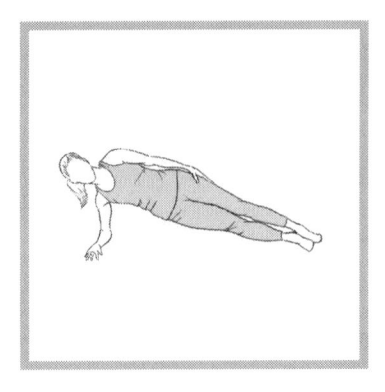

Once you have completed both sides, move on to the next exercise.

Side Plank up and Down

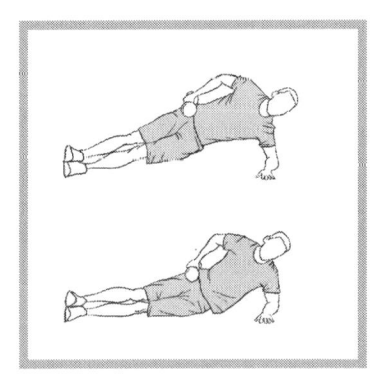

This exercise should be done for 30 seconds on each side.

- Position yourself on your side with your forearm flat on the floor and your elbow directly under your

shoulder. Extend both legs with your feet stacked on top of each other.
- Lift your hips off the floor so that your body is straight. Place your opposite hand on your hip or alternatively raise your arm in the air.
- Lower your hip toward the ground, as close to the ground as possible.
- Lift your hip back into the starting position.
- Repeat this exercise for 30 seconds.

Once complete, move on to your other side and repeat the exercise. When you have done both sides, move on to the next exercise.

Side Plank Reach Through

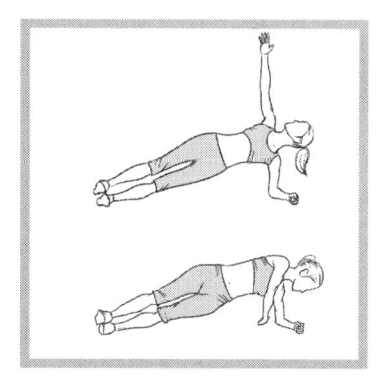

This exercise should be done with 30 seconds on each side.

- Position yourself on your side with your forearm flat on the floor and your elbow directly under your shoulder. Extend both legs with your feet stacked on top of each other.
- Lift your hips off the floor so that your body is straight.
- Bring your opposite arm through the space between your body and the floor. Twist your chest as you do this. Reach as far back as possible.
- Retract your arm and chest back to the starting position.

Once complete, repeat the exercise on your other side. When you have completed the exercise on both sides, move on to the next exercise.

Mountain Climbers

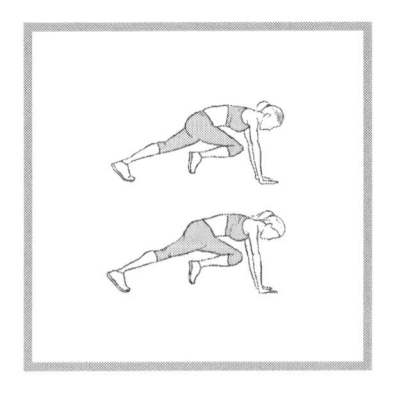

Complete thirty repetitions of this exercise. Fifteen repetitions on each side.

- Position yourself on the floor with your legs extended behind you and your arms extended in front of you. Place your palms flat on the floor.
- Bring one knee up into your chest without compromising your form.
- Switch your legs and repeat using the other leg. Switching should take place simultaneously so that your legs are always moving.
- Do this exercise as fast as possible without compromising your form.

Once you have completed this exercise, move on to the next and final exercise.

Bicycle Crunches

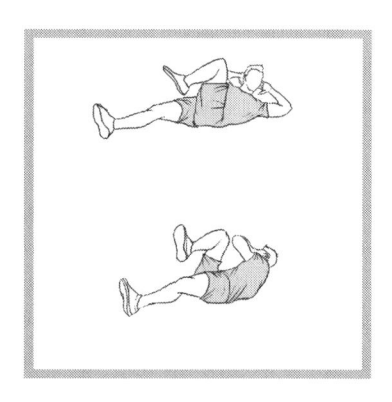

This exercise should be done for thirty repetitions, fifteen repetitions for each side.

- Lie flat on the floor and place your hands behind your head.
- Lift your legs slightly, keeping them extended. Raise your back slightly off the floor.
- Bending one leg toward your chest, bring the opposite elbow to your knee while keeping the other leg extended and raised off the floor. You will need to twist your upper body slightly to achieve this motion.
- Move your leg back into the starting position while simultaneously completing the same movement using the opposite leg and arm.

Once you have completed this exercise, repeat the entire workout another three times. You may wish to add rest periods in between exercises, but little to no rest is recommended. 30-60 seconds of rest may be incorporated after each circuit.

LEG WORKOUT

This exercise is recommended by the Calisthenic Movement (2019, 03:15–05:21) to help develop and strengthen your legs. This workout should be done as a giant set, meaning that there is only one set of each exercise, and there should be no rest in between exercises. Each exercise should be done until you are fatigued. To move this workout to a more advanced level, you can add weight to each workout.

Pistol Squat

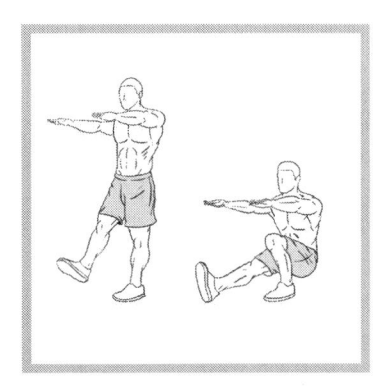

Do this exercise until you feel fatigued. You can add weight to make the exercise more challenging. It is recommended that you start with your weaker leg, as this exercise will become more difficult the second time around.

- Stand on one leg with your toes pointed forward.
- Extend one leg in front of you, keeping it as straight as possible.
- With all your weight on one foot, slowly sit into a squat. Keep your other leg extended and elevated.

- Use your grounded leg to push yourself up into the starting position.

Repeat this exercise until you feel fatigued. Once fatigued, alternate your legs and start again.

If you cannot yet do the pistol squat, you may do assisted pistol squats. Assisted pistol squats follow the same steps as the pistol squats, but you can hold on to something for support and to help you maintain your balance.

You can also do the pistol squats on a raised platform to make the exercise easier, as it does not require you to keep the opposite leg as elevated as in traditional pistol squats.

If this is still too difficult, you can do a slow step up. To do the slow step up, you will need a platform of at least knee height.

- Stand facing the platform. Put your hands on your hips and place one foot on top of the platform.
- Slowly, straighten your leg to raise yourself toward the platform. Lean forward slightly to maintain your balance.
- Once your leg is completely straightened, proceed to lower yourself back into the starting position.
- Repeat the exercise.

Once you become fatigued using one leg, alternate your legs and start again.

Archer Squat

This exercise should be done until you experience fatigue.

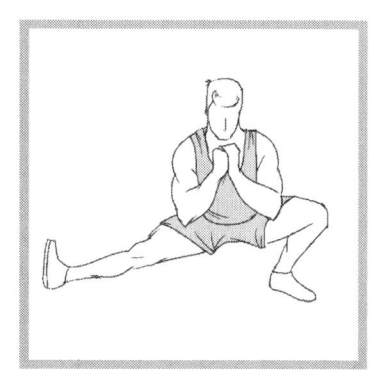

- Stand with your feet in a wide stance. Position your legs far enough to allow you to squat as deeply as possible. Position your feet facing outward.
- Shift your weight onto one leg. Lean your hips backward and bend your leg toward the floor while extending the other, and move into a sitting position.

- Pause with your knee over your toes and your leg parallel to the floor. Do not move your knees beyond your toes.
- Using your bent leg, push yourself back into the starting position.
- Repeat the exercise with the opposite leg.

It is essential to keep your heels on the ground throughout the exercise.

Glute-Bridge

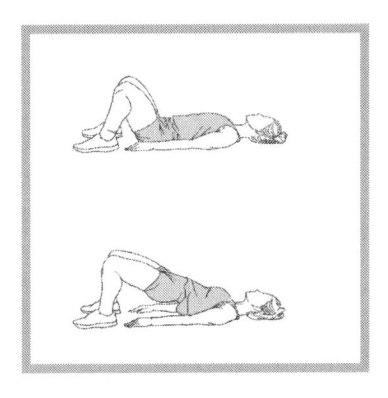

Do this exercise until you experience fatigue and feel you cannot continue.

- Lay down with your back on the floor, knees bent, and feet flat on the floor. Note that the more bent your knees are, the easier the exercise will be.

- Extend both of your legs. To make harder extend one leg.
- Without using your hands, push your hips off the ground into an elevated position until your spine is straight.
- Slowly lower yourself back into the starting position.

Once fatigued, repeat this exercise using the other leg until fatigued.

Jumping Lunges

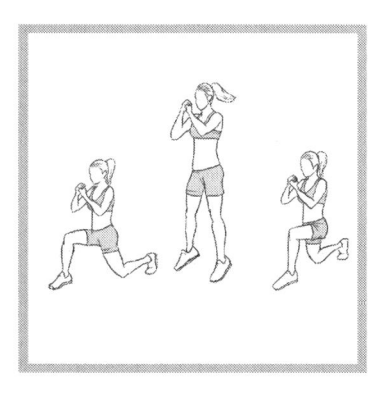

This exercise is a cardiovascular exercise, so some exertion is expected. Try to do the exercise until your legs are fatigued, rather than focusing on your breathing.

- Stand with your feet approximately shoulder-width

apart.
- Take a big step forward with your right leg and shift your weight onto that leg.
- Now, bend your right leg to lower your body until your leg is parallel to the floor. Your opposite leg may also be bent toward the ground so that your shin is parallel to the floor.
- Jump up and switch your legs, so your left leg is now bearing your bodyweight, and the right leg is bent downward.
- Repeat the exercise.

For an easier alternative, you can do regular lunges. This exercise is similar, but much less exertive and less cardio-intense.

- Stand with your feet approximately shoulder-width apart.
- Take a big step forward with your right leg and shift your weight onto that leg.
- Now, bend your right leg to lower your body until your leg is parallel to the floor. Your opposite leg may also be bent toward the ground so that your shin is parallel to the floor.
- Slowly, using your leg, push yourself up into the starting position, keeping your back straight.

- Alternate your legs and repeat the exercise.

This exercise should be done until fatigued.

Deep Squat Hold

Do this exercise until your leg muscles are fatigued.

- Stand with your feet approximately shoulder-width apart and your toes pointing outwards.
- Lean your hips backward, bend your legs toward the floor, and move into a sitting position. Keep your chest up and shift your weight to your heels.
- Squat as low as you can manage and hold that position. Your squat should be deeper than your knees.
- Once you have reached the deep squat position, hold for as long as you can manage. Be sure to keep your heels on the ground throughout the exercise.

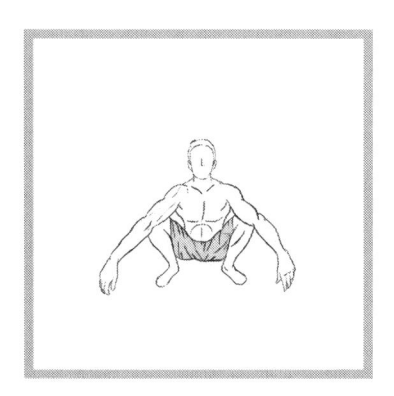

Alternatively, you can squat to your lowest possible position and hold it there.

Another more recommended alternative is an assisted deep squat hold. This requires you to go as deep as the deep squat, but with assistance from a bar, wall, or bench. Use an object to help you get to the deep squat position and maintain your balance.

Single-Leg Calf Raises

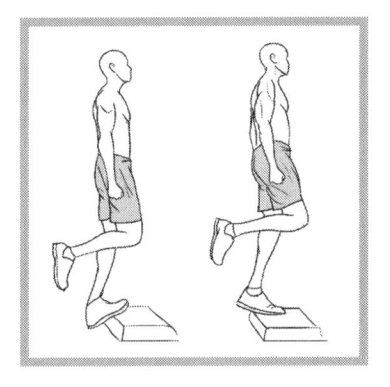

This exercise is best performed on a raised platform for optimal results. Make sure that you have something to hold on to, to help you maintain your balance. Do this exercise to the point of fatigue.

- Stand with the ball of your foot on the raised platform, and the other leg raised off the floor. Place your hand on the wall or hold on to something to balance yourself.
- Lift the heel of your foot as high as you can manage, squeezing your calves.
- Lower your heel back to the starting position.
- Once the first leg is fatigued, switch to your other leg.

Once the exercise is completed, your workout is complete.

These workouts are a great way to start your split workout routine if you are unfamiliar with the principles of such a routine. From here, the exercises can be amended and changed according to your needs and goals. You can decide to adopt a circuit routine or complete the workout in sets. Rest periods, sets, and repetitions can be adjusted according to your level and your exercise goals.

7

ADAPTION - MISTAKES YOU CAN AVOID

Seeing Calisthenic professionals and experts on YouTube can be inspiring and can have you attempting to execute rather strenuous and complicated exercises and tricks right away. You forget, however, that mastery takes a significant amount of time and patience. These professionals and experts have probably been doing Calisthenics for years. Executing these exercises correctly requires perfect form and the mastery of numerous progressions along with the basic Calisthenic movements. There are several commonly held misconceptions about Calisthenics that leave people with little or no progress, injuries, and frustration. People try to jump the gun on these exercises and end up jeopardizing their own progress.

Addressing these misconceptions and mistakes will help you to avoid making them and prevent you from believing in these myths as you construct and follow your Calisthenic routine. Injuries often accompany these mistakes, and more often than not, these are back, shoulder, or wrist injuries. Being aware of these common injuries and how to manage and prevent them will save you from unnecessary injury and strain.

COMMON MISTAKES

There are many mistakes that people frequently make when it comes to Calisthenics and misconceptions that they pick up along the way. Misinformation can be dangerous and detrimental to your Calisthenic journey and your level of progress. Take note of these mistakes and learn from them so you can avoid having to make them all yourself.

1. Favoring muscles over movements.

Since weight training generally focuses on developing one muscle or group of muscles at a time, people often attempt to apply the same principle to Calisthenics. They may plan a workout session with a specific focus on the arms, legs, or core, for example. As I have mentioned previously, however, Calisthenic exercises are compound and work more than one muscle at a time. Trying to isolate certain muscles will not work with Calisthenics. Instead, plan your workout around certain movements such as push or pull movements and focus on the movement. Allow the exercise to do what it needs to do and to engage the muscles that it should be engaging.

2. Jumping the gun.

Seeing the experts do a human flag or muscle-up on YouTube can be very inspiring, as it should be. Most people make a mistake, however, of jumping the gun and attempting these complex movements right off the bat. These exercises take time and cannot merely be done overnight. Mastering these exercises consist of countless progressions, as well as a mastery of the basic Calisthenic exercises. Start your journey by mastering the more basic exercises first before attempting more complex exercises. Be realistic about your skill and ability level. This is the only way to reach your ultimate goal.

3. Favoring quantity over quality.

As I have mentioned previously, quality is more important than quantity in Calisthenics. Being able to do thirty reps of push-ups is worthless if these movements are rushed and done without the proper form. It is more effective to do fewer reps using the correct form. If you are unable to execute an exercise as it should be done, attempt a progressive approach, mastering easier movements first and working your way up to the real thing. There is no shame in having to do an easier variation of an exercise first. On the contrary, starting with these movements will become a stepping stone to better performance, increased strength, and perfect execution.

4. Half-measures.

People often make the mistake of not allowing full range of motion when doing exercises. Not going low enough when you do a push-up, for example, or not squatting deep enough. They would rather attempt half a push-up than opt for the knee push-up. By not allowing full range of motion in your exercises, you are robbing yourself of the full benefits of the exercise. Again, do fewer reps of simpler progressions and focus on your form rather than limiting the fruits of your labor. These progressions are designed and intended to strengthen the muscles needed to execute the real thing.

5. Unrealistic goal setting or even no goal setting.

As I have explained in Chapter 4, goal setting is essential when you exercise. Not only does it determine the kind of exercises you should be doing, but it also keeps you motivated and helps you keep track of your progress. It is important to be realistic in our goal setting. Expecting yourself to do a full muscle-up by the end of the month when you've never even done a chin-up is unrealistic and will set you up for failure. Unrealistic goal setting can be demotivating and frustrating. It is essential, to be honest with yourself. That being said, you should focus on setting both long-term and short-term goals. If your long-term goal is to be able to do a full-on muscle up, concentrate your short-term goals on mastering the chin-up first, then the pull-up, and so on. Celebrating your milestones significantly increases your motivation and sense of achievement.

6. Focusing only on your strength areas.

Some people neglect their areas of weakness entirely and shift their focus to their areas of strength instead. By doing so, you are robbing yourself of the benefits that you can reap with Calisthenics. Remember Bob, the builder in Chapter 4? Ignoring your weak areas will crumble your foundations, making you even weaker in those areas. Rather than ignoring these areas, spend some time developing them and turn them into strengths. Developing your weaknesses as well as your strengths, will give you a well-rounded set of skills instead of limiting the exercises that you can do.

7. Comparison.

There is a reason that they call comparison the thief of joy. Comparing yourself to professionals and experts in the field is unrealistic and detrimental. Those professionals have had months, possibly years, of training. Be gracious with yourself and allow yourself the time and the space to develop your skills without the unnecessary added pressure. Rather, use these professionals as someone to look up to and their skills as something to look forward to as you progress.

8. Improper form or technique.

Improper form is the primary cause of injury and the single most common cause of slow or no progress. Having the correct form is vital to reap the maximum benefits of Calisthenic exercises (or any exercises for that matter). Progressions and variations are designed to isolate certain movements from the exercise and help you develop the appropriate form. Mastering the correct form is the most challenging part of learning a new exercise. Once you have mastered the correct form, executing the exercise should be much easier, and progression is just a matter of strength.

9. Assuming progress is linear.

Most people assume that progress is linear, and beginners often expect to see results almost instantaneously. These expectations are unrealistic. More often, progress is exponential, meaning that the longer you exercise, the more likely you are to see more and more progressive results. Consistency and determination are key aspects. When it feels like you are getting nowhere, and you feel like giving up - keep pushing. You will soon break through the proverbial wall and see the hard-earned fruits of your labor.

10. Not training the lower body.

This is something that Calisthenics are often mocked for and is true in a number of cases. You may have seen the jokes about skipping leg day at the gym. A number of people, especially men, tend to focus only on developing and strengthening their upper body. They focus mainly on exercising the abs, shoulders, back, and arms, and neglect their lower body as a result. Not only is this unattractive, but it is also very unhealthy and places unnecessary weight and strain on your lower body.

11. Not warming up.

The majority of injuries, sprains, and pains are caused by neglecting to warm up. I have mentioned the importance of warming up in Chapter 1 of this book. Muscles that are warmed up are less likely to be strained and injured. Warming up is not only an exercise for beginners. Athletes, experts, and professionals acknowledge the importance of warming up. Don't allow something as trivial as not warming up to keep you from achieving your goals.

12. Fixed routines.

Unlike weight training, Calisthenics does not require fixed and repetitive routines. Varying your exercises and progressions is beneficial to your progress, in fact. Using the same, repetitive routines will stagnate your process and leave you in a rut. Once you are comfortable with an exercise or routine, that means it's time to change it up. Use more complex progressions of exercises and change up your routine by increasing repetitions and sets or changing the order of the exercises. This keeps the body from getting too used to any exercise or routine and getting stuck in a rut. Practicing the same routine every day puts your body at risk of falling into a habit and stalls your progression.

COMMON INJURIES

The most common injuries in Calisthenics are back, shoulder, and wrist injuries. The three main causes of injuries in Calisthenics are improper form, overtraining, and overloading. By understanding these three causes and how they contribute to injury, you will be able to avoid these common injuries and improve your Calisthenic training.

I have highlighted the importance of form countless times already, and I emphasize it again. In Calisthenics, quality is always more important than quantity. When you execute your exercises, pay attention to your form and make sure that you can execute these correctly. Use easier variations and progressions to help you develop the correct form and execution. Once you can master the correct form, you will be able to learn exercises more easily, and you will see a significant increase in your strength and development.

Overtraining causes your body to become weaker rather than stronger. The most common signs of overtraining include persistent fatigue and muscle pain, an elevated resting heart rate, loss of motivation, insomnia, and decreased appetite. Overtraining occurs when you do not provide your body with enough rest or nutrition to recover effectively after a workout. Cutting down your rest time and food intake in an effort to achieve results more rapidly can be detrimental and will eventually lead to stagnation or even regression in strength.

Overloading occurs when you put your body under more weight and strain than it can endure. Luckily Calisthenics only loads your bodyweight most of the time, which your muscles are designed to support, but overloading can still be a problem. A progressive increase in intensity and complexity is essential. Progressions are beneficial because they allow the body to develop and increase its strength gradually. Avoid putting your body under too much strain by applying gradual progressions rather than leaping into more taxing and complex exercises.

Several strategies can be applied to avoid unnecessary strains and pains. Firstly, always warm-up before you exercise. Warming up the muscles prepares your body for exercise and prevents unnecessary strain. Cardiovascular exercises are good warm-up exercises to get your heart pumping and your blood flowing. Stretching is another strategy that will significantly reduce the risk of injury. Stretching increases your flexibility and range of motion, as well as the blood flow to your muscles. Focus on your form and technique when you perform exercises. Make use of progressions to help you perfect your form. Lastly, provide your body with enough rest and recovery time to prevent overtraining and keep your body functioning at the optimal level.

THE IMPORTANCE OF STRETCHING

Stretching before and after a workout is an excellent way to avoid injury. There are countless benefits to stretching, both for your training and your overall health.

1. Prevent injury:

Stretching helps to prevent injury while training. By lengthening your muscles, you will reduce muscle stiffness and consequently reduce the chances of injury.

2. Improved blood flow:

Improved oxygen flow is another advantage of stretching. This helps your body circulate blood more easily, therefore warming up your muscles and keeping you energized. This factor also helps to reduce fatigue both generally and during exercise by keeping the body and mind alert.

3. Enhanced performance:

Stretching helps you to perform better in your exercises. Warm muscles, increased blood flow, and raised energy levels are all factors that can significantly improve your performance—stretching increases both your motivation and energy, helping you develop an unbreakable mindset.

4. Muscle repair:

Stretching after a workout can speed up muscle repair and prevent stiffness and injury. It also protects your joints, as it significantly reduces the pressure in the joints. By bringing down your heart rate and cooling down your body, it also prevents dizziness and nausea.

5. Increased range of movement:

I have already discussed how important range of movement can be in training. Stretching improves flexibility and therefore leaves you with a greater range of movement. This will directly affect your training results.

6. Remedies back and neck pain:

Stretching is known to both heal and prevent back and neck pain, as it releases muscle tension. It also helps you develop a better posture, which will be beneficial in the long run.

When you start stretching for the first time, it is crucial, like anything else, to start slow. Your body needs to get used to the exercises and movements, especially if your body is inflexible. Pay attention to your form and technique, as this will affect the results of your stretches.

Natasha Freutel (2019) suggests the following stretch routine for beginners. This routine is short, easy to do, and requires no equipment. It also covers the entire body, making it a good routine to start with. You should see significant improvement in your flexibility and performance in no time. Then you should move on to more targeted and comprehensive stretching routines.

Knights Stretch

This exercise stretches the lower body. This stretch should be repeated for both sides.

- Stand with your feet about shoulder-width apart.
- Step back with one leg and place your hands on the floor on either side of your foot.
- Lower your hips and hold. You should feel a stretch your hip and leg. Hold this position for 30 seconds.
- Now extend your front leg as far as possible while keeping your hands on the floor. Hold this position for 30 seconds.

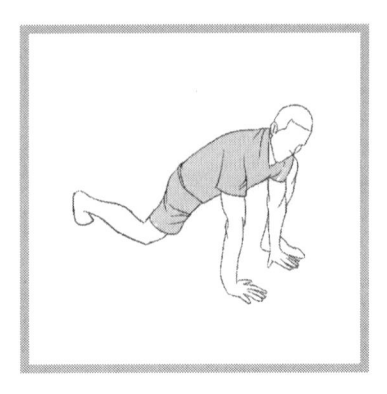

Repeat this stretch on the other side.

Forward Fold

This stretch is a full-body stretch that focuses on the shoulders, hamstrings, lower back, and chest.

- Stand with your feet approximately shoulder-width apart and join your hands behind your glutes by interlacing your fingers.
- Bend at the waist, shifting your hips backward and placing the weight on your heels. You should feel the stretch in the back of your legs.
- You can pull your arms up above your head while you bend forward, going as far as your shoulders can manage.
- Hold this position for 30 seconds.

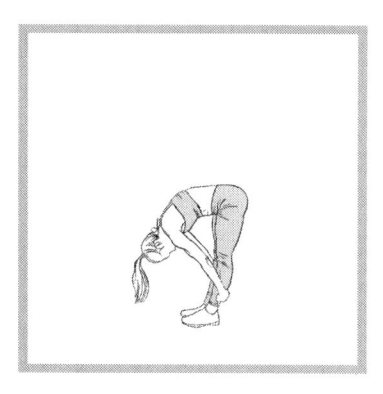

Once you have relaxed your muscles, you can repeat the stretch.

Seated Piriformis Stretch

This stretch is useful for relieving back pain and improving mobility. This stretch is not recommended for persons with back problems or prior surgeries.

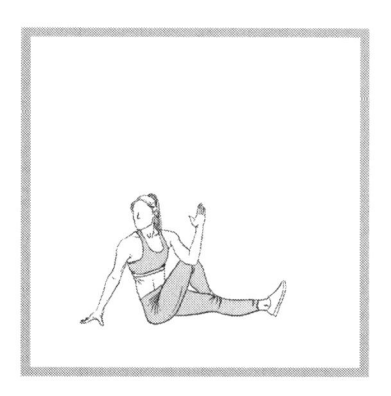

- Sit on the floor with your right leg crossed over the left one, which is out straight in front of you.
- Twist your shoulder toward the right. Push against your right leg for support.
- Pull this stretch as far as you can manage, hold for 30 seconds, and release.

Repeat the stretch on the right side.

Reclining Bound Angle

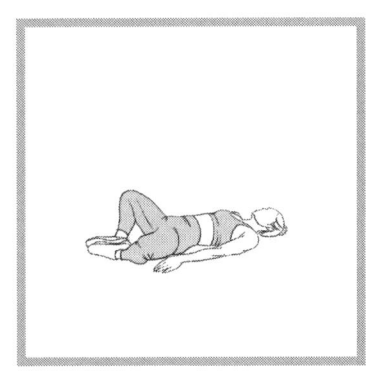

This stretch focuses on releasing tension in the hips and inner thighs.

- Sit on the floor with your back straight and the soles of your feet touching.
- Place your hands on your knees and straighten your spine.

- Keeping your back straight, with each exhale bring your knees closer to the ground.
- Stretch as far as you can manage and hold the stretch for 30 seconds.

As you do this stretch, try to get your head closer and closer to your feet, until you can touch your feet with your head.

Wall Chest Stretch

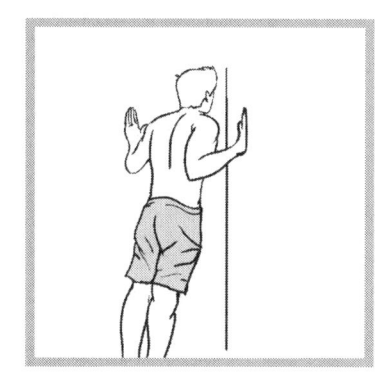

This exercise helps to improve posture, breathing, and focuses mostly on the chest and some parts of the arms.

- Stand in the center of an open door and place your forearms on either side of the doorframe. If this is not possible, stretch one arm at a time.
- Keeping your forearms on the doorframe, lean

forward until you feel a stretch in your chest and shoulders.
- Go as far as possible and hold for 30 seconds.

This is a good stretching routine to start with. Once you are more comfortable with these stretches, you can attempt other stretches and even design your own stretching routine suited to your needs. As you progress, you will find yourself becoming more flexible and therefore increasing your range of motion significantly. Stretching is so important that there is too much to cover all in this book. It can make a huge difference not just in your workouts but also in your quality of life.

8

OPTIMIZATION - THE LIFESTYLE YOU SHOULD AIM FOR

Calisthenics is not merely another exercise approach that you can use to develop your strength. Calisthenics is a lifestyle, and like all lifestyles, it will require some significant changes and include many sacrifices. Calisthenics is something that you should commit to consistently. The most important lifestyle factors that need to be adapted are sleep, diet, and consistency. Focusing on these three factors and adjusting them correctly will help you to receive the maximum benefits from Calisthenics and live a healthy life. Altering these factors will improve not only your physical health but your mental health as well.

SLEEP

Surprisingly, sleep is an essential part of a healthy and active lifestyle. Developing healthy sleeping habits will significantly improve your physical and mental health and will dramatically improve your exercise regimen. Sleeping helps your body to recover, preserve energy, and repair muscles that were affected during exercise. It is also while we are asleep that our body produces growth hormone. This hormone is what helps the body build, repair, and grow muscle. Studies show that adults need between seven and eight hours of sleep every night to function optimally.

Not only is getting enough sleep beneficial to your exercise routine, but a lack of sleep can significantly impact your ability to exercise. Sleep deprivation can make your workouts feel harder and more challenging. Those who experience sleep deprivation are more likely to feel fatigued much quicker than they usually would. A lack of sleep will, therefore, negatively affect your exercise and can contribute to overtraining syndrome.

While getting enough sleep is beneficial to your exercise regimen, the reverse is also true. Exercise has been proven to help people fall asleep more easily, experience deeper sleep, and feel less restlessness during the night. Sleep and exercise are, therefore, intimately connected and are in a direct relationship with one another.

Sleep is not only crucial for an active lifestyle, however. Sleep is also a key factor in overall health and body function. Studies indicate that poor sleeping habits are directly linked to weight gain and obesity. Getting enough sleep regulates your appetite and keeps you from overeating and developing an unhealthy appetite. Furthermore, quality sleep improves cognitive functioning and affects concentration and memory. Sleeping is also proven to reduce health risks significantly and can improve your immune function. Insufficient sleep can lead to depression and temperamental emotions, while quality sleep can decrease moodiness and improve the ability to read others' emotions - an essential social skill.

Sleeping is, therefore, not only beneficial to your exercise regimen but helps to promote an overall healthy lifestyle.

DIET

Keeping a healthy, balanced diet is not only good for your health. It will also support your new Calisthenic lifestyle and significantly improve the benefits gained from your new healthy habits. The concept of dieting is often unhealthy and unsustainable. Developing and keeping healthy eating habits is more sustainable and is more likely to benefit you in the long run. There are several dietary strategies to consider that will help you to live healthier and optimize your new lifestyle. It is vital to take note of the kinds of food you consume and be mindful of what these foods contribute to your overall functioning.

Proteins

Proteins are essential for body growth and maintenance. They are integral in muscle-building and repair. They, therefore, provide us with the energy we need to get through the day and complete our daily tasks. Proteins can be found in poultry, red meats, fish, dairy, legumes, and eggs. Lean proteins are recommended for healthier intake, and red meats and processed meats should be limited as they can be fattening. Although most people tend to include protein in dinner meals and some lunches, proteins should also be included in breakfast meals. They should be consumed and portioned throughout the day.

Fruit and Vegetables

Fruits and vegetables are rich in fiber, minerals, and vitamins, among other things. Their low-fat content and calorie count make them one of the healthier dietary options. Fruits and vegetables of different sorts and colors contain various vitamins, minerals, and antioxidants. You should, therefore, eat a variety of fruits and vegetables to ensure that you are providing your body with all the necessary vitamins, minerals, and antioxidants. Dried fruit and raw vegetables are great alternatives for a snack during the day. Try adding a fruit or vegetable to every meal you eat. This, combined with snacking, will increase your fruit and vegetable intake significantly and provide your body with the nutrients it needs to function effectively.

Fats

Despite popular opinion, fats are not necessarily taboo in a healthy diet. Fats are another source of energy. Certain fats can help to reduce inflammation and provide calories that can fuel your workouts. Fats also contribute to keeping your hair and skin healthy. Unsaturated fats are healthier than saturated fats and help provide essential fatty acids and calories that keep the body active and moving. These healthy, unsaturated fats can be found in nuts, seeds, avocados, olives, and oils. Olive oil is a healthy option.

Workout Foods

Fueling up before and after a workout requires a balance of carbohydrates and protein. This combination can help you feel more energized during your workouts. Some simple workout snacks include bananas, berries, grapes, oranges, nuts, and peanut butter. These foods can help fuel your workout and provide you with enough energy to get through your workout more efficiently. Not only do they fuel your workouts, but they also accelerate the recovery process, helping you to come back bigger and stronger much sooner. Michael Roussel, a bodyweight training expert, suggests eating within two hours of your workout to optimize the benefits of the workout (Gaddour, 2014, p. 18). He further indicates that carbohydrates are best to consume after a workout to adjust your sugar levels. Proteins are also good foods to consume after a workout to increase muscle-building speed. Whey protein shakes are an excellent way to consume protein after a workout.

Calories

Despite popular belief, it's also not good to cut too many calories from your diet. Often when people want to lose weight, this is the first thing they do. While cutting calories can speed up the weight loss process, your calories shouldn't be reduced too much. A lack of calories can leave you feeling tired or ill, and that's not healthy. Calories provide the body with the energy it needs.

Calories are your friend. You need to use them to control your goals. Make sure to consume a healthy balanced diet without skipping any staple meal. Focus on increasing calories in those major meals or in beneficial healthy snacks. If you are trying to gain muscle or strength, you need 15%

more than your sustaining calorie level; in this case, carbs can be your friend, although try and avoid refined carbs. If you aim to burn fat, then focus on increasing your heart rate and the intensity of the workout, take out the snacks and make sure to increase the proportions of protein in your diet these are all proven ways to lose weight and burn fat.

If the body takes in more calories than it uses, those calories will result in weight gain, this can be beneficial if you want to build muscle, but you need to make sure it's the right foods. If you eat fewer calories than you burn, then you will lose weight, but make sure that you don't starve your body because you do not want to lose that muscle too.

Beverages

Substituting your regular soda for a diet soda simply won't do the trick. Studies suggest that diet soda is no better than regular soda and may even lead to increased health risks. Most people would then opt for fruit juice as a substitute for soda. Studies suggest, however, that fruit juice is equally high in sugar and can contribute to weight gain. Due to the lack of fiber present in fruit juices, eating the fruit would be the healthier option.

On the other hand, fruit juice is rich in vitamins and minerals that can be healthy. Therefore, fruit juice does have some health benefits. When purchasing fruit juice, look for brands that are 100% fruit juice and contain no added sugar. Most fruit juices are artificial and provide little or no value compared to the actual fruit. Fruit juice should, therefore, be consumed in minimal quantities, if at all. If you do love fruit juice, limit yourself to one glass per day. Be careful, though! The majority of fruit juices that are sold in grocery stores are watered-down, artificial versions of the good stuff.

Drinking water is an underrated dietary strategy that holds countless benefits. Studies show that drinking water can aid the weight loss process by speeding up the metabolism. Studies also show that an increase in water intake may be directly linked to a decreased calorie intake because water contributes to regulating the appetite. Furthermore, drinking more water will leave you feeling energized and alert. There is absolutely no harm in drinking water - it contains zero calories!

Balance

A balanced diet is a fundamental part of a healthy diet. Listen to your body; it will tell you what it needs. An important thing to note is not to skip breakfast. Breakfast is an essential part of your day and sets your digestive system in motion. Skipping breakfast will be to your own detriment as you will for sure feel a crash later in the day. If you are trying to build muscle, then breakfast is extra important as your body has not been fed energy in 8 hours; breakfast will stop those gains from being eaten up.

Maintaining a healthy diet on a tight schedule can be difficult, but many strategies can help you to stay healthy without compromising your busy schedule.

First off, plan your breakfast in advance. As I have said before - do not skip breakfast! Even on a tight schedule, it is possible - and healthy - to still have breakfast. Even if you are looking to lose weight, breakfast is important. You do not want to feel tired during the day; instead, try eating breakfast later. Initiating a window from brunch to dinner 11 am-7 pm, which is the only time you can eat, can increase the amount of time your body is in its fasting mode. This is the basic premise of intermittent fasting as your body entering fasting mode reduces insulin and increases the growth hormone; this is associated with easier fat burning.

Breakfast smoothies are one of the most efficient breakfast choices, as they are easy to consume on-the-go. Pre-pack your smoothie ingredients so you can simply pour it, add a liquid base such as milk, yogurt or juice, blend it and go. You can even add a scoop or two of protein powder to boost your energy and your workouts. If these are not to your taste, overnight oats are another healthy and quick breakfast option. Pre-pack your oats with whatever layers you want to add (fruit, seeds, honey), add milk and refrigerate overnight. In the morning, you can simply grab your breakfast and go.

Secondly, plan your snacking. Those snack cravings are an inevitability, and merely hoping that you won't get them is unrealistic and unwise. Rather than hoping for the best, plan ahead. Keep some healthy snacks around your office, in your car, and at home to prevent yourself from stopping for a quick chocolate bar or a pack of chips when you crave a snack. Nuts, yogurt, fruit, and raw vegetables are ideal healthy and nutritious snacks to keep around. These snacks can be a fantastic way to contribute to your calorie intake if you are looking to build muscle.

Meal preparation is your friend. Plan your lunches beforehand, and make sure they are ready to grab-and-go on your way to work. This will not only help you to stay healthy but will also help you save money by cutting on lunch expenses. Some healthy ideas for lunch include salads, healthy sandwiches using wholemeal bread or fruits and vegetables. Wraps are also a very healthy and delicious option for lunch.

Plan your dinners ahead of time. You want to make sure you have a well-balanced meal planned for every night of the week, a quarter protein, a quarter carbs, and half veg is a great place to start; try to add minimal dairy. A meal like vegetable and chicken fried rice or grilled salmon and creamy mash with roasted vegetables is a perfect combination of these food groups. There are innumerable ways to do this. With certain foods like casseroles, you can cook these beforehand and freeze them. When you get home, you can simply microwave them or heat them in the oven if you do not have time to cook. Add some vegetables to your meal and enjoy. Alternatively, plan your meals and make sure that you have all the ingredients you need. When you get home, you can simply look at the schedule and cook whatever it is that you had planned. Meal planning helps you ensure that you are getting enough vitamins and minerals. Meanwhile, meal preparation reduces the time it takes to cook and prepare meals, thereby saving you a significant amount of hassle.

CONSISTENCY

As the saying goes, consistency is key. Consistency must be practiced in all areas in order to reap the maximum benefits of Calisthenics. This means practicing consistency in your exercise routine, your diet, and your sleeping patterns. By practicing consistency in these areas, you will end up constructing healthy habits, making it much easier to live an active and healthy lifestyle. Patience is a virtue when it comes to healthy living. You might not see the benefits and outcomes of these immediately, but you'll receive double the rewards later if you pass them up now. As Dawn Graham once said: "Lifetime regrets are more painful than delayed gratification" (Goodreads, n.d.-b). Don't substitute delayed gratification for lifetime regret.

Exercising only when you feel like it will get you nowhere. I'm not saying you should exercise all day, every day. To gain the most out of your exercise, you will need to set up an exercise routine. Use the strategies discussed in Chapter 4 to create your own realistic routine, suited to your needs - and stick to it! Exercise should become a habit, and habits take time to develop. If you've just started exercising, chances are you'll feel super motivated for the first day or two. Maybe you're a real enthusiast, and you manage to maintain your motivation for the first week. You will, however, experience a time where the motivation runs dry, and you might not feel like exercising. This is exactly when you need to stick to your planned routine.

Practice the art of self-discipline and follow your routine regardless of whether you've had a hard or busy day. Be deliberate about carving time out in your busy schedule for exercise. Rather than settling for "sometime today" or "later today," set a specific time and duration for your workout every day and commit to doing your workout during that time. Being vague about your workout schedule will likely lead to procrastination and postponement. Before you know it, it's 9 pm, and you still haven't completed your exercise for the day. Being deliberate about scheduling your workouts will prevent procrastination and help you to stay motivated and disciplined in your exercise. Keeping a consistent routine will also benefit you physically, helping you to build your endurance, strength, and muscle at a faster, more consistent rate.

The same kind of consistency applies to your diet and nutrition. Being consistent and disciplined in your dietary habits will significantly improve your exercise and notably accelerate your progress. There is no use in eating healthy for three days and then rewarding yourself by binge eating junk food and treats. Being consistent and deliberate about your diet is the first step to being healthy. It's okay to indulge now and again, but make sure these are planned or scheduled to avoid overindulging and consequently reversing all the benefits you've worked so hard to achieve.

One strategy that you can apply to help you practice consistency is to plan your weekly meals ahead of time. Keep a journal or schedule in which you outline the meals that you plan to eat for breakfast, lunch, and dinner every day. In doing so, you can buy the necessary ingredients over the weekend or when you have time, and avoid the last-minute rush of finding something to eat when you get home after a long, hard day. Planning your meals and making sure you have the ingredients to make those meals will help you to avoid grabbing something quick and artificial or opting for the drive-through.

Keeping a food journal is another way to keep track of what you've eaten and be more conscious about what goes into your body. You'd be surprised by the amount of unhealthy snacking you do throughout the day. Keeping a food journal will help you keep track of your food intake and will raise your awareness of how much and what you eat throughout the day. Some things you may consider including in your food journal are what you eat, the portion size, time of intake, place, hunger level at the time, and how you are feeling at the time. Emotions and external factors have a surprising effect on your eating habits, and keeping track of these factors at the time of intake might help you to identify those factors that trigger unhealthy eating habits or cravings.

Having a consistent sleep schedule is the third and final cog in the consistency machine. Keeping a regular sleep schedule has many scientifically proven health benefits. Some of these have already been discussed earlier in the chapter. Having a set bedtime or bedtime routine helps our bodies anticipate what is coming and therefore prepares us for sleep. This anticipation improves our quality of sleep and leaves us feeling well-rested in the morning. Furthermore, science proves that not getting enough sleep increases the risk of dying earlier. Getting enough sleep will help to maintain the balance in your body's hormones, which improves your mood and even helps you lose weight. Regular sleep also increases your alertness and levels of energy, which increases your productivity and engagement significantly. Regular sleep also helps to restore and repair the body's skin and muscle tissue, helping your muscles recover after a workout. As an added benefit, getting enough sleep improves your body's coordination - definitely something you can use to enhance your Calisthenic performance.

As mentioned above, having a regular bedtime routine can significantly improve the quality of your sleep. It does so by conditioning your brain to identify when it is time to sleep. If you follow the same routine before bed every night, your brain will begin to recognize those behaviors and will, therefore, prepare itself to sleep once you start the routine. This will significantly reduce the time it takes to fall asleep and provide you with more restful sleep. Your bedtime routine should include reducing screen time and doing something that you find relaxing. These activities may consist of reading, stretching, meditation or prayer, or taking a long, warm bath. Engaging in calming activities before bed will help your brain to power down and reduce the number of racing thoughts and ideas that may arise while you sleep. Keeping a regular bedtime routine also conditions your body's internal clock and helps you to fall asleep faster and wake up more easily.

BUILDING HEALTHY HABITS

Healthy living starts with building healthy habits. They say that it takes 21 days to form a habit - that is, twenty-one days of commitment and dedication. Once you have reached the twenty-one-day mark, consistency should be much easier to practice. There are, however, some steps that need to be followed when developing a habit.

1. Pick a starting point.

What is it you want to achieve? Decide on a healthy habit you want to foster in your life - be it healthy eating, sticking to your exercise routine, or establishing a consistent sleeping pattern. Pick one goal that you feel is the most urgent.

2. Find a solution.

How are you planning to go about reaching the goal you have just identified? Think about what is holding you back from eating healthy, sticking to your exercise routine, or keeping a consistent sleeping routine. Find realistic solutions to these problems.

3. Make a plan.

Devise a strategy to overcome these challenges and start developing those habits. Ask yourself what you need to achieve these goals. If you need to buy some healthy groceries, some new equipment, or a new bedside alarm, go ahead. These will also motivate you and get you excited about starting your new, healthy habits.

Set up a schedule for yourself and stick to it. If you need to, buy an exercise tracker, a sleep tracker, or a food journal to help you keep track of your new habits. These are all ways to keep you motivated and excited.

4. Put your plan into action.

Once you have devised a plan, start! This seems like an obvious one, but so many people spend so much of their time planning to be better and to do better, but they never get around to doing it. Don't spend all your time on planning and devising, put your plan into action.

5. Reward yourself.

Finally, it is essential to reward yourself for doing well and sticking to it. By this, I don't mean rewarding yourself with an entire tub of ice cream because you've eaten well during the week. Think of rewards that you will enjoy without jeopardizing your progress. Plan a trip or buy something you have wanted for a while now. Spoiling yourself with something that will boost your motivation is even better - a new gym outfit, new equipment, a brand new water bottle, or some comfortable slippers. Don't let your reward be something that keeps you from achieving your goal.

Being healthy is not merely about improving your Calisthenics. There are innumerable reasons for maintaining a healthy lifestyle, and an improved mental health state is one of these benefits. Having healthy exercise, eating, and sleeping habits has innumerable benefits that will improve your mental health and help you avoid excessive mood swings, depression, and unnecessary stress.

The purpose of Calisthenics does not start and end with working out. Calisthenics will leave you feeling - and looking - great!

FREE WORKOUT PLANNER & KILLER CORE WORKOUT

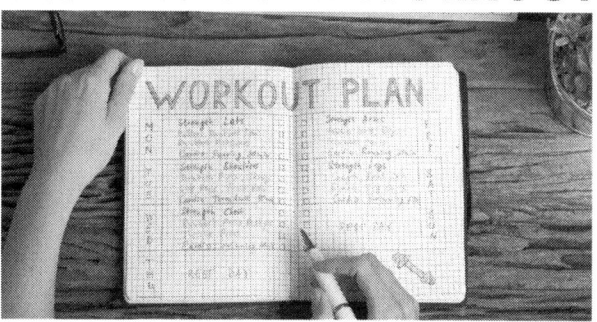

Want to make sure you reach your fitness goals?....you won't without tracking your progress! and did you know most exercises depend on a strong core for results?

1. Get your FREE perfect workout planner.
2. Get my FREE killer core workout so you reach your goals faster
3. Simply print off or download onto your device
4. And feel amazing as you watch your progress skyrocket

to receive just type in the following link :).......

https://fitnessmilo.activehosted.com/f/1

YOUR MISSION SHOULD YOU CHOOSE TO ACCEPT IT…….

I need your help; I am new to publishing and working my socks off day and night to try and bring you the best content in my books.

So, your mission from me is that if you enjoyed the book, leave me a quick and honest review. So we can get my books seen by more people and let them know the quality of my books, this is top secret information and we are running out of time

P.S. if you did not enjoy the book, instead of leaving a negative review please contact me letting me know why you did not like the content and I will do my best to address your concerns

Thank you :)

CONCLUSION

This book has proven that Calisthenics is an effective and efficient exercise approach that has countless benefits. Anyone at any level can start Calisthenics, and even the most gravity-defying exercises can be mastered with the right attitude and exercise routine. Calisthenics can easily be done in the convenience of your own home and in your own time, making it the most efficient and practical exercise solution. By focusing on bodyweight alone, Calisthenics reduces the amount of strain on your muscles and joints and increases your control over your body. This aspect also makes Calisthenics one of the most accessible exercise approaches. Calisthenics is the perfect solution for those who have hectic schedules and busy lives.

By mastering the basic movements and exercises of Calisthenics, you will already have your foot in the door. Once

CONCLUSION

you have mastered the foundational push, pull, leg, and core exercises, you will be equipped to move on to more intense and complex exercises. There are easier exercises and progressions, to begin with, that will help you focus on your form and execution, since these are crucial in the field of Calisthenics. Progressions are an excellent strategy to help you develop the necessary strength and form to execute exercises effectively. A good approach to start your first exercise routine is to start with a full-body routine consisting of basic push, pull, leg, and core exercises. Starting each exercise with the highest progression, you can manage, work your way down to the easiest progression. This will help you to develop your endurance and strength while simultaneously improving your form and execution.

Once you have mastered the basics and can perform every progression with perfect execution, you can then move on to constructing your very own Calisthenics workout routine. The most important factors to note here are setting goals, identifying your weaknesses, determining the frequency of exercises, rest, intensity and volume, and tempo. These factors are an essential foundation for any exercise routine and will determine the structure and nature of your exercise routine. Your goals will determine the direction of your exercise routine. While your long-term goals will inevitably determine the direction of your macro-cycle, you should also set short-term goals that will fuel your micro-cycles and keep you motivated.

Each workout should focus on developing a range of motion, skill, and strength. These are the three critical aspects of Calisthenic exercises. Your goals and abilities will determine the type of workout you will adopt. Although full-body workouts are recommended, split workouts can help you to achieve specific movements and exercises more effectively by focusing on either specific movements or specific muscle groups.

While the idea is appealing, you cannot simply dive in and start attempting the most taxing and complicated exercises. This idea is merely one of many commonly held misconceptions that you need to take note of in your Calisthenic journey. It is imperative that you understand these misconceptions and that you know the truth about them. Being aware of these will help you to avoid common mistakes and assumptions made by others in the field and thus avoid setbacks in your progress. The most common and frequent injuries are back, shoulder, and wrist injuries. These injuries most often occur due to inconsistent form and execution. Practicing progressions will help you to avoid these injuries.

Moving between progressions can take time, depending on your ability and skill level. Skills and strength are not merely

CONCLUSION

developed overnight and can take months to master. Overtraining and overloading are the other most common causes of injuries. Other strategies that you can apply to prevent these injuries from occurring include stretching and ensuring that you get ample rest. Having a regular stretching routine is very important and beneficial to your exercise regimen, as it increases your range of motion and performance levels. Stretch at least once daily to improve your flexibility, exercise performance and range of motion, and your overall well-being. Keeping a sleep journal and developing a nighttime routine will help you to get more and better quality rest. This will also be beneficial to your exercise regimen.

It is important to note that Calisthenics is a lifestyle, which means that some major lifestyle changes should accompany it. Sleep, diet, and consistency are the three key factors in constructing a healthy lifestyle. The Sleep Advisor (2020) provides some shocking statistics relating to sleep and sleeping habits:

- According to the Centers for Disease Control and Prevention, 35% of adults sleep less than the recommended seven hours per day.
- The National Center for Biotechnology Information reports that more than a hundred

thousand deaths can be attributed to medical complications caused by sleep deprivation.
- They also indicate that nearly 20% of motor vehicle accidents and injuries are related to sleepiness and sleep deprivation.
- Harvard School of Public Health highlighted that 3-5% of obesity in adults might be attributed to sleep deprivation.

Getting enough quality sleep is therefore crucially important, both to your own well-being and the well-being of those around you. The amount and quality of sleep that you clock every night can have a direct impact on your exercise regimen and your overall health. Sleep and exercise are shown to be directly linked. To get the most out of your new Calisthenic lifestyle, make sure that you are getting the necessary seven to eight hours of sleep every night. Having a regular bedtime routine can help you to improve your sleep quality and condition your internal clock.

Nutrition is another essential factor that directly impacts your exercise regimen and progress. Dieting is not a sustainable solution. By being conscious of your eating and drinking patterns, you will ensure that you receive the maximum benefits from your exercise routine and improve your rate of progress. Keep a food journal to help you keep track of your food intake. This

CONCLUSION

will help you to be more aware of your eating habits and motivate you to maintain a healthier diet. Planning your weekly meals can also help you to maintain a healthy and balanced diet.

Lastly, consistency is key. This is true of your workout routine, your sleeping habits, and your diet. Be mindful and deliberate when you plan your meals and exercises, and be sure to carve out specific times in your schedule for your exercises. Make exercise and healthy nutrition a habit rather than a spur-of-the-moment, instantaneous fix. Don't allow your desire for instant gratification to get in the way of your long-term progress. Delayed gratification might be challenging to accept, but it will benefit you more in the long run.

If this book did not convince you to start exercising regularly, Med Alert Help (Hrubenja, 2020) provides some statistics that will hopefully encourage you to get moving and active and make some lifestyle changes.

- Physical exercise is said to lower the risk of heart disease by more than 20% and decrease the risk of dementia by 30%.
- Shockingly, the World Health Organization reports a 20% to 30% increased risk of death among people who do not exercise regularly, making a lack of exercise one of the leading risk

factors for an increased death rate on a global scale.

- The World Health Organization recommends that adults between the ages of 18 and 64 years should have at least one hundred and fifty minutes of moderate exercise per week, or seventy-five minutes of intense exercise per week.
- The World Health Organization also reports that physical inactivity is more prevalent in high-income countries. This could be due to the increasingly demanding nature of the corporate world.

This is why Calisthenics is a sustainable exercise solution. It allows you to exercise anytime without needing any equipment. Your workout routines can be kept at short, but intense intervals, providing you with enough exercise to stay healthy without jeopardizing your career or your busy schedule. By keeping an exercise schedule and a sleep and food journal, you will be able to keep track of your well-being more effectively while still adhering to your demanding schedule. By applying the strategies discussed in this book, you will save yourself significant amounts of hassle and time.

In this book, I have provided you with everything you need to start and sustain your Calisthenic journey. I have

CONCLUSION

provided you with an explanation of what Calisthenics is, and I have highlighted some of the benefits of choosing Calisthenics over other forms of exercise. I have given you all the necessary steps to do the most basic Calisthenic exercises, as well as the more complicated and progressive variations of these exercises. I have provided you with a beginner workout plan covering all the basic exercises and movements that you can use to start your Calisthenic journey, and I have provided you with the tools to construct your own effective and realistic workout routine.

I've also given you several programs and progressions that will help you to master the most complicated and aesthetic Calisthenic exercises. I have helped you understand the difference between full-body workouts and split workouts, and I have provided you with some examples of split workout routines, both for a circuit approach and when using sets to get you started. I have educated you on the most common mistakes and injuries made in the field of Calisthenics, as well as some strategies for avoiding these mistakes and injuries. Finally, I have provided you with all the tools you need to turn Calisthenics into a lifestyle by monitoring your sleep and diet and practicing consistency in all aspects of your lifestyle.

If all of this has sparked your interest in Calisthenics and you wish to find out more, there are countless blogs, vlogs, and

YouTube videos to help compliment this book. Chris Heria from THENX (n.d.) has countless very valuable tutorials, recommendations, and videos on how to complete certain exercises and workouts proficiently. He has a number of videos on progressions and variations, too, if you are still struggling with form. He also has a blog and posts various vlogs on YouTube that are related to Calisthenics. Other organizations like Saturno Movement and Calisthenic Movement offer tutorial videos on exercises and tips on how to complete certain exercises, mistakes to avoid, etc. You can also refer to the reference section for some of the other sources I have used in this book. You have a world of information at your fingertips.

With all the knowledge and tools at your disposal, the onus is now on you. Take these tools, tips, and trades and apply them to your life. People often say that knowledge is power, but that sentiment is not true. It is as Rob Liano has said: "Knowledge on its own is nothing, but the application of useful knowledge, now that is powerful" (Goodreads, n.d.-a). I have given you a mountain of useful and actionable knowledge that will help you to start your Calisthenic journey. I have provided you with countless solutions, strategies, and factors to consider that will significantly ease this journey.

I have equipped you to develop and lead a healthy lifestyle, providing you with practical solutions and strategies to

CONCLUSION

apply on the course of your journey. I have shown you all that you need to know to design and effectively execute your very own Calisthenic exercise program—using either a split or full-body routine to achieve that movie star physique. I have gone above and beyond by supplying you with a simplified version of scientific research and providing you with several workout examples that you can follow or model in creating your own exercise regimen. It is now up to you to take all you have learned in this book and turn it into something powerful and life-transforming.

I have taken your hand and led you straight to the proverbial watering well. I have done my best to fill it to the brim, but I cannot make you drink it. It is up to you whether you will drink from the well or succumb to thirst. I hope you choose a healthy, exciting life filled with all that Calisthenics can offer you. Whichever option you choose, I wish you the best of luck!

REFERENCES

A. (n.d.-a). What Are The Basic Calisthenics Exercises? Retrieved May 11, 2020, from https://improvephysique.com/what-are-the-basic-calisthenics-exercises/

Adidas Runtastic Team. (2018, December 4). Customize Your Training with Exercise Variations (EASIER & HARDER). Retrieved May 16, 2020, from https://www.runtastic.com/blog/en/bodyweight-exercise-variations/#8_Leg_Raises

Ash and Em. (n.d.-b). How To Build Healthy Habits. Retrieved June 6, 2020, from http://www.simpleluxeliving.com/build-healthy-habits/

Axe, J. (2018, May 11). The Dangers of Soda: Why Regular and Diet Are So Bad for You. Retrieved May 15, 2020, from

REFERENCES

https://www.runtastic.com/blog/en/diet-soda-vs-regular-soda/

AZ Quotes. (n.d.). Malcolm X Quote. Retrieved May 16, 2020, from https://www.azquotes.com/quote/184510?ref=knowledge-is-power

Beast, B. (2019, January 6). 5 Most Common Calisthenics Mistakes – Bine Beast. Retrieved May 15, 2020, from https://www.binebeast.com/2019/01/06/5-most-common-calisthenics-mistakes/

Bouchez, C. (2009, October 2). Doing the Perfect Push-up. Retrieved May 12, 2020, from https://www.webmd.com/fitness-exercise/features/doing-the-perfect-push-up#3

Calisthenic Movement. (n.d.). Cali Move. Retrieved June 8, 2020, from https://www.calimove.com/

Calisthenicmovement. (2019, April 26). Say NO to Chicken Legs! | Bodyweight Leg Workout | [Video file]. In YouTube. Retrieved from https://www.youtube.com/watch?v=-AOpemH7Tb4

Carter, J. (2019, March 8). Calisthenics Or Weights – What Should You Pick. Retrieved May 10, 2020, from https://www.gearhungry.com/calisthenics-vs-weights/

Chertoff, J. (2018, June 7). What Are the Benefits of Flutter Kicks and How Do You Safely Do Them? Retrieved June 6,

2020, from https://www.healthline.com/health/fitness-exercise/flutter-kicks#safety

Chertoff, J. (2020, June 22). What Are the Benefits and Risks of Doing Daily Pushups? Retrieved May 12, 2020, from https://www.healthline.com/health/fitness-exercise/pushups-everyday#how-to

CHRIS HERIA VLOGS. (2019, March 28). MY FAVORITE 6 PACK ABS WORKOUT FOR FAST RESULTS + NUTRITION [Video file]. In YouTube. Retrieved from https://www.youtube.com/watch?v=RqxgO13OXkI&t=466s

Cirino, E. (2017, April 25). 8 Calisthenics Exercises for Beginners. Retrieved May 11, 2020, from https://www.healthline.com/health/fitness-exercise/calisthenics#whatsthe-difference

Cronkleton, E. (2019, October 24). Tone Your Core, Shoulders, and Hips with a Russian Twist. Retrieved June 4, 2020, from https://www.healthline.com/health/russian-twist#instructions

Davies, D. (2018, November 9). The complete guide to calisthenics. Retrieved May 11, 2020, from https://www.menshealth.com/uk/building-muscle/a759641/complete-guide-to-calisthenics-everything-you-need-to-know/

REFERENCES

Dips. (n.d.). Retrieved May 12, 2020, from https://www.calisthenicexercise.com/dips/

Drayer, L. C. (2017, April 7). Is fruit juice healthy? Retrieved May 16, 2020, from https://edition.cnn.com/2017/04/07/health/is-fruit-juice-healthy-food-drayer/index.html

Eastman, H. (2018, February 28). The Ultimate Beginner's Guide To Calisthenics. Retrieved May 11, 2020, from https://www.bodybuilding.com/content/the-ultimate-beginners-guide-to-calisthenics.html

Eating Healthy on a Tight Schedule. (2017, May 30). Retrieved June 7, 2020, from https://medikeeper.com/blog/eating-healthy-on-a-tight-schedule/

Freutel, N. (2019, November 12). A Daily 5-Minute Stretching Routine That Everyone Needs. Retrieved June 4, 2020, from https://www.healthline.com/health/fitness-exercise/daily-stretching-routine

Gaddour, B. (2014). Men's Health Your Body is Your Barbell: No Gym. Just Gravity. Build a Leaner, Stronger, More Muscular You in 28 Days! (1st ed.). New York, United States of America: Rodale Books.

Get Healthy U. (n.d.). How to Do Mountain Climbers. Retrieved June 8, 2020, from https://gethealthyu.com/exercise/mountainclimbers/

REFERENCES

Goodreads. (n.d.-a). A quote by Rob Liano. Retrieved May 15, 2020, from https://www.goodreads.com/quotes/643023-knowledge-is-power-no-knowledge-on-its-own-is-nothing

Goodreads. (n.d.-b). Lifetime Regrets Quotes (1 quote). Retrieved May 16, 2020, from https://www.goodreads.com/quotes/tag/lifetime-regrets

H. (2017a, February 7). Learn how to master pistol squats with this progression template. Retrieved June 6, 2020, from https://fits-me.co/pistol-squats-progression/

Halse, H. (2019, July 31). 9 Stepup Variations for Leg Strength and Power | Fitness | MyFitnessPal. Retrieved June 5, 2020, from https://blog.myfitnesspal.com/9-stepup-variations-for-leg-strength-and-power/

Higgins, C. (2019, January 7). Dynamic Stretching and Warm-up for Calisthenics. Retrieved June 6, 2020, from https://www.calisthenics-gear.com/stretching-warm-up-calisthenics/

How To Front Lever: The Complete Beginner's Guide. (n.d.). Retrieved May 15, 2020, from https://www.morethanlifting.com/how-to-front-lever-the-complete-beginners-guide/

Howcast. (2012, July 31). How to Do Leg Flutters or Flutter

REFERENCES

Kicks | Sexy Legs Workout [Video file]. In YouTube. Retrieved from https://www.youtube.com/watch?v=eEG9uXjx4vQ

Hoyles Fitness. (2012, September 15). The Physiology of Muscle Building. Retrieved May 15, 2020, from https://www.hoylesfitness.com/physiology/the-physiology-of-muscle-building/

Hrubenja, A. (2020, January 19). 30 Exercise Statistics & Facts That Will Get You Moving! Retrieved June 8, 2020, from https://medalerthelp.org/exercise-statistics/

Hundson, J. (n.d.). The Ultimate List for Common Strength Training Mistakes to Avoid. Retrieved May 16, 2020, from https://www.lifehack.org/articles/lifestyle/the-ultimate-list-for-common-strength-training-mistakes-to-avoid.html

Jackson, D. (n.d.). Programming for Calisthenics. Retrieved May 17, 2020, from https://schoolofcalisthenics.com/2017/06/24/programming-for-calisthenics/

Kavadlo, A. (2012, March 2). How to Perform the Human Flag | T Nation. Retrieved May 15, 2020, from https://www.t-nation.com/training/how-to-perform-the-human-flag

Kavadlo, A. (2017, January 1). Human Flag Tutorial: Steps to

REFERENCES

Achieve the Human Flag. Retrieved May 15, 2020, from https://gmb.io/human-flag/

Kilroy, D. S. (2019, February 21). Eating the Right Foods for Exercise. Retrieved May 15, 2020, from https://www.healthline.com/health/fitness-exercise-eating-healthy#calories

Lindberg, S. (2018, June 8). Stretching: 9 Benefits, Plus Safety Tips and How to Start. Retrieved June 6, 2020, from https://www.healthline.com/health/benefits-of-stretching

Lindberg, S. (2019a, May 30). How to Do Jumping Lunges. Retrieved June 6, 2020, from https://www.healthline.com/health/jumping-lunges#how-to-do-it

Lindberg, S. (2019b, July 25). How to Do a Muscle Up on Bars and on Rings. Retrieved May 15, 2020, from https://www.healthline.com/health/how-to-do-a-muscle-up#muscles-at-work

Lindberg, S. (2020, March 11). Stretching: 9 Benefits, Plus Safety Tips and How to Start. Retrieved May 12, 2020, from https://www.healthline.com/health/benefits-of-stretching#benefits

Lyda, J. (2020a, April 22). Calisthenics For Beginners (9 Key Workouts + More). Retrieved May 11, 2020, from https://athleticmuscle.net/calisthenics-for-beginners/

REFERENCES

Lyda, J. (2020b, April 22). The Benefits of Calisthenics: 8 Reasons To Do Bodyweight Workouts. Retrieved May 10, 2020, from https://athleticmuscle.net/benefits-of-calisthenics/

M. (2019, August 15). The iron cross progression: Full guide from beginner to gymnast. Retrieved May 16, 2020, from http://www.mastersofbodyweight.com/how-to-iron-cross-a-complete-guide-from-beginner-to-master

Mace, D. (2015, July 10). 12 Rules for Gaining Strength. Retrieved June 5, 2020, from https://www.mpcalisthenics.com/strength-training/12-rules-for-gaining-strength

Marcin, A. (2019, May 23). How to Do Chair Dips. Retrieved May 10, 2020, from https://www.healthline.com/health/chair-dips#how-to-do

Mazzo, L. (2019, June 14). What Is Calisthenics (and Should You Be Doing It)? Retrieved May 10, 2020, from https://www.shape.com/fitness/trends/what-is-calisthenics-workout-benefits

Medvesek, H. (2019, February 18). Squats: What Proper Squats Look Like & Which Muscles They Work. Retrieved May 12, 2020, from https://www.runtastic.com/blog/en/squat-4-common-squat-mistakes-avoid/

Michael & Yannick. (2019, October 1). Calisthenics Pull

REFERENCES

Workout Example. Retrieved May 11, 2020, from https://calisthenics-family.com/articles/calisthenics-pull-workout/

OFFICIALTHENX. (2017a, July 17). Calisthenics VS Weights | THENX [Video file]. In YouTube. Retrieved from https://www.youtube.com/watch?v=nmP8l-ELI3Q

OFFICIALTHENX. (2017b, April 3). How To Start Calisthenics - L SIT & PISTOL SQUATS | THENX [Video file]. In YouTube. Retrieved from https://www.youtube.com/watch?v=flQVCWBuVgk&list=PLX8QIwhN83ZXbP19JNDn8_usq5_2uJ3gL&index=3

OFFICIALTHENX. (2017c, March 20). How To Start Calisthenics - PULL UPS | THENX [Video file]. In YouTube. Retrieved from https://www.youtube.com/watch?v=tB3X4TjTIes&list=PLX8QIwhN83ZXbP19JNDn8_usq5_2uJ3gL&index=1

OFFICIALTHENX. (2017d, April 10). Start Calisthenics with This Workout | THENX [Video file]. Retrieved from https://www.youtube.com/watch?v=kIVxdIWy7Eo&list=PLX8QIwhN83ZXbP19JNDn8_usq5_2uJ3gL&index=4

OFFICIALTHENX. (2018, October 1). Benefits of Calisthenics [Video file]. In YouTube. Retrieved from https://www.youtube.com/watch?v=92w3RCjl2S4&list=PLX8QIwhN83ZXbP19JNDn8_usq5_2uJ3gL&index=5

REFERENCES

Openfit. (2020, March 24). How to Do the Single-Leg Calf Raise. Retrieved June 5, 2020, from https://www.openfit.com/how-to-do-single-leg-calf-raise

Pace Kinetics. (n.d.). Full Body vs.Split Workout Routine, Which One Is The Best For You? Retrieved June 4, 2020, from https://pacekinetics.com/full-body-vs-split-workout-routines-best/

Perry, M. (2019, December 25). Full Body Workout Vs. Split Routine: Which Is Better? Retrieved June 5, 2020, from https://www.builtlean.com/2011/09/15/full-body-workout-vs-split-routine-which-is-better/

Quinn, E. (2020a, March 4). How to Do a Bicycle Crunch. Retrieved June 6, 2020, from https://www.verywellfit.com/bicycle-crunch-exercise-3120058

Quinn, E. (2020b, April 11). How to Do Pushups: Proper Form, Variations, and Common Mistakes. Retrieved May 12, 2020, from https://www.verywellfit.com/the-push-up-exercise-3120574

R. (2017b, December 11). A Complete List of Calisthenics Exercises. Retrieved May 10, 2020, from https://www.calisthenics-101.co.uk/a-complete-list-of-calisthenics-exercises

Richling, C. (n.d.). The Benefits of a Food Journal. Retrieved

May 12, 2020, from https://www.ornish.com/zine/proven-benefits-keeping-food-journal/

Saturno Movement. (n.d.). Saturno Movement. Retrieved June 8, 2020, from https://saturnomovement.com/

SaturnoMovement. (2018a, October 17). Full Body Workouts VS Split Training in Calisthenics (HOW DO I TRAIN?) [Video file]. In YouTube. Retrieved from https://www.youtube.com/watch?v=nS6bqzlETgI

SaturnoMovement. (2018b, November 21). PULL Workout Calisthenics Routine For ALL LEVELS (Follow Along) [Video file]. In YouTube. Retrieved from https://www.youtube.com/watch?v=xWs67ToUgjA&t=1008s

SaturnoMovement. (2018c, November 28). PUSH Workout Calisthenics Routine For ALL LEVELS (Follow Along) [Video file]. In YouTube. Retrieved from https://www.youtube.com/watch?v=t1JRBoeRAvI&t=337s

Schultz, R. (2019, February 8). How To Do A Side Plank Flawlessly. Retrieved June 6, 2020, from https://www.womenshealthmag.com/fitness/a20697895/basic-workout-side-plank/

Silberman, L. (n.d.). Build Endurance and Stamina With These Tactics. Retrieved June 4, 2020, from https://www.

REFERENCES

mensjournal.com/health-fitness/build-endurance-and-stamina-with-these-exercises/

The Sleep Advisor. (2020a, January). 54 Shocking Sleep Statistics, Data and Trends Revealed for 2020. Retrieved June 7, 2020, from https://www.sleepadvisor.org/sleep-statistics/

The Sleep Advisor. (2020b, June 3). 54 Shocking Sleep Statistics, Data and Trends Revealed for 2020. Retrieved June 7, 2020, from https://www.sleepadvisor.org/sleep-statistics/

THENX. (n.d.). Thenx. Retrieved June 8, 2020, from https://thenx.com/

Top 8 Calisthenics Exercises to get you started! (2018, May 26). Retrieved May 11, 2020, from https://www.pullup-dip.com/calisthenics-exercises

Tucker, A. (2016, September 9). How To Do Boat Pose, A Mat Exercise For Your Abs. Retrieved June 5, 2020, from https://www.self.com/story/this-mat-exercise-will-transform-your-core

Willis, J. (2017, June 4). 6 Row Machine Alternatives to Give Your Body an Amazing Workout. Retrieved June 5, 2020, from https://www.gq.com/story/row-exercise-alternatives

USE IT OR LOSE IT

STRETCHING EXERCISES TO REGAIN AND MAINTAIN YOUR OPTIMUM FLEXIBILITY

<u>FREE</u> WORKOUT PLANNER & KILLER CORE WORKOUT

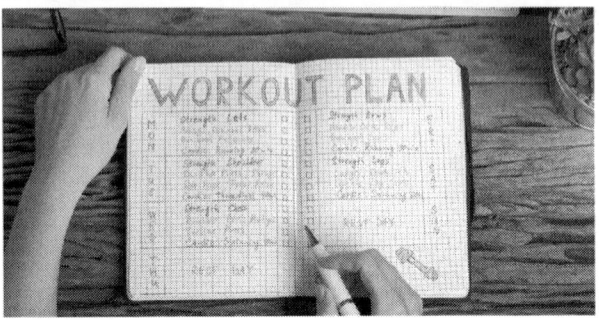

Want to make sure you reach your fitness goals?....you won't without tracking your progress! and did you know most exercises depend on a strong core for results?

---

1. *Get your FREE perfect workout planner.*
2. *Get my FREE killer core workout so you reach your goals faster*
3. *Simply print off or download onto your device*
4. *And feel amazing as you watch your progress skyrocket*

---

to receive just type in the following link :).......

https://fitnessmilo.activehosted.com/f/1

INTRODUCTION

Many people of all ages suffer from stiffness and mobility issues. Movement is at the base of being alive; we can't get away from it, which is why it is so important to be able to do it with ease. When people suffer from persistent stiff muscles or pain during movement, they usually attribute it to age, injury, or something else that they cannot control. Maybe those things can play a factor, but lack of flexibility is the number one cause of stiff muscles and pain.

If you suffer from constant injuries while training, hindered movement due to muscle stiffness, or pain, then you may have a flexibility issue. The good news is that you do not have to suffer from this forever; flexibility is something that you can gain over time. What you need is a tailor-made set of stretches and flexibility exercises that will help you increase your mobility. Not all stretches are created equal,

INTRODUCTION

and some only work for specific needs and circumstances, that is why just doing generic stretches will not work. The road to flexibility and increased mobility is a journey that you need to be guided along so that you can get the best out of it.

After years of experience as a personal trainer and physio, I have confronted every reason for inflexibility in the book. Because of this, I have been able to devise tailored solutions to various problems. I take pride in my ability to help people along this journey and am confident that I will be able to help you. Being able to reach a place where your body can have its full range of motion with no pain or stiffness is life-altering. All it takes is a few simple routines and consistency, and I know you will be able to reach the level of flexibility you once were and even exceed that.

My clients are now enjoying their lives much more; they did not know how free life could be until they were able to remove the constraints that their bodies had. They are much happier, and they can reach their fitness goals much quicker, training is no longer a chore but rather a joy to do. With a little effort, you can also have a similar story. You will be able to touch your toes with ease, walk for hours with no pain, and take your training to the next level. Movement will no longer be an obstacle that is standing in your way, but the stepping stone you can use to reach your other goals.

INTRODUCTION

This book will be filled with routines, tips, tricks, and knowledge I have passed on to my clients, who are now enjoying life to the full. They now know that nothing can stand in their way. They can push themselves more each day because they see what their bodies are capable of. Once they reached this realization, they became more confident in their bodies' capabilities, and that is what I want for everyone who reads through these pages.

By the time you are done with this book, you will be fully equipped with the knowledge that will help you gain back your flexibility or tap into the flexibility you never knew you had. Armed with stretches and routines that have been tailor-made for your circumstance means that you get to focus on what is best for you. It will cut out the frustration of trying lots of different things that just don't work. Everyone's body and circumstances are different, and that is why I have made sure that there is something for everyone in this book.

Until you make an effort to start working on your flexibility, stiff and sore muscles will always be an issue. In fact, the longer you do not address the problem, the worse it will get. Flexibility is not only about excelling in sports and fitness but also in your everyday life. Inflexibility can get in the way of doing simple tasks like bending down to fetch something from the cupboard or picking up your child or grandchild.

INTRODUCTION

The sooner you start, the sooner you can begin reaping the benefits. You will feel younger and be able to perform the tasks that now cause a problem, with ease.

The knowledge that I will be passing on to you has helped hundreds of people. They now live more nimble and pain-free lives, all because of the guidance provided in this book. Each chapter will provide you with the steps and support needed to make the most out of your potential mobility and say goodbye to your flexibility struggles. Applying what you learn will lead you to improve flexibility problems associated with pain and stiffness, so you no longer have to deal with it daily. Once you start feeling and seeing the results from utilizing the tools given to you in this book, you will never look back.

Your better, freer, and more mobile life is just on the other side of these pages. Once you start unlocking the potential that your body has, you will want to push forward and try new things. My goal is that everyone who reads this book will benefit in some way and, as a result, live a better life altogether. If you want to lose the inflexibility chains that have bound you for so long, then this is your first step. Let's go on this journey together.

1

THE WARM-UP: BENEFITS OF STRETCHING THAT YOU ARE MISSING OUT ON

Stretching is often overlooked when planning a workout program. Usually, people have goals like losing weight or gaining muscle, and they believe that stretching will not be of much help to them. This kind of thinking is incorrect; stretching is vital to every movement of your body. It allows your body to have the freedom to move as it pleases and reduces the amount of pain you will have when exerting pressure on your muscles.

THE IMPORTANCE OF STRETCHING

Stretching is not only a physical thing, but it also overflows in every part of your wellbeing. It will increase the level in which your body can move, improve your quality of life, even impact your mental wellbeing. It is what will empower your body to do the activities that will help you reach your body goals and can be used as a tool to calm your mind through life's ups and downs. What's even more impressive is that's just scratching the surface of how beneficial stretching can be to your life.

Exercise

Stretching is focused on lengthening the muscles, and it allows your muscles to function better. When you stretch, it improves your body's mobility, which is so essential to exercising. When you exercise, you are using your muscles, that's why you need them to be in top form. Increasing your range of mobility will benefit the way you exercise because you will not be restricted to tight muscles, you will be able to engage more muscles in your body and increase the quality of your workout.

Flexibility is sometimes not thought of as something linked to strength. This is entirely false, and if you don't believe me, just look at people who do yoga, both men and women alike have toned bodies and a significant amount of strength. Flexibility in itself is not strength training, but because your muscles work together in everything, you are able to get more out of your strength workouts when you are more flexible.

Stretching is not a warm-up, as we have popularly thought. The truth is that you will get better results from stretching if your muscles are already warmed up. The best thing you can do is do a quick five-minute jog or walk around the block to get your muscles moving, then begin stretching. Your muscles will be looser, and you will get more out of your stretching routine. If you would like you can move on to your other exercises, your muscles will be nice and limber. When we incorporate stretching into our routine, it almost guarantees a reduction in injuries when exercising or putting any strain on our muscles. Our muscles are less likely to seize up and move into different positions more easily.

General Living

The lives we live now are quite sedentary, meaning that we don't move around a lot. We end up sitting at desks for most of the day, the most mobile part of our body is our fingers which are typing away at the keyboard. This isn't good for our muscles; in fact, sitting on a chair for most of the day will definitely result in tighter hamstrings. Now I am not saying you have to quit your job and become a professional athlete to be healthy, but balance is needed to keep your body healthy.

This balance is found when incorporating stretching into your routine. Sometimes we get so caught up in our busy everyday routine that we forget to do what is good for us. If you have ever suffered from stiff joints and pain or stiffness in certain muscles, even when you don't remember doing anything that can cause that feeling, then you should know that this is a direct result of a lack of mobility in your muscles.

Mobility will help you to go about your daily tasks with ease. Not being able to bend down to get something from the floor or a low shelf because of stiff muscles is not the greatest feeling, and it gets in the way of you just living your life. A high-quality life is one with as little restrictions as possible, we all want the freedom to do as we please, and our bodies should not be the thing that holds us back from doing that. This is precisely why flexibility and mobility are essential.

As we get older, our muscles and joints naturally get stiffer. Increasing your flexibility by stretching actually slows down this process. Getting started today will have you saying thank you in the future. We all still want to be able to do the things that we enjoy; we don't want aging to stop us from enjoying our lives. The earlier you start, the better it will be for you. However, don't discount the benefits of stretching in older years, stretching will always have massive benefits for whoever does it, regardless of age.

A direct result of stretching is healthier and stronger

muscles. When our muscles are strong, our posture also improves. Slouching is a common problem today, and it can cause pain in your neck and back, and in severe cases, it can even lead to fatigue and shortness of breath. When we stretch, it encourages the proper alignment of our muscles, which pulls our bodies up and reduces the risk of slouching and bad posture.

Another benefit of stretching is that it increases the blood circulation in our bodies. That means our bodies will be able to function better because of the increased blood supply to our muscles. With the increase in blood supply comes an increase in nutrients; this means the nutrient supply to our muscles is increased. You will also experience less soreness because of this increased blood and nutrient supply in your body. Your body will be able to function better as a whole.

Mental Wellbeing

During the day, our minds are so busy, always having problems to fix or a crisis to tend to. It is difficult to take the time to gather your thoughts and just focus on you. Not having time to clear your mind and focus on something that calms you can have negative impacts on your mental state. When you are always on the move, there is no time for rest, and we all need rest to perform our best. This rest should be both a physical as well as mental rest; we often overlook the latter.

When we stretch, it is a series of slow, controlled movements. We are forced to focus on ourselves, what our bodies are doing, and how we are feeling. This gives your mind a mental break from all the thoughts that are continually running through your mind. You have time to give your mind a break, destress, and begin to catch up with your thoughts. When you are done, you will feel more ready to take on the next set of challenges.

We can carry tension in our muscles; you will notice this in knots in your muscles, especially around your neck and shoulders. It is a defensive strategy used by our bodies when we are feeling stressed or overwhelmed. This can affect your performance throughout the day; you will be feeling uncomfortable and will always be thinking about the tension you are carrying in your muscles. Stretching provides a better outlet for this stress, not only that it can help with preventing knots in the future.

Stress and tension have a negative effect on our mental wellbeing. What goes on in our minds will eventually overflow into all other areas of life. Don't overlook how important mental health is to your overall health and happiness. We need to take care of all aspects of our wellbeing.

DO IT RIGHT

As much as it is important to start somewhere, we have to be doing things correctly. Granted, you will not be an expert at the beginning of this journey, but neglecting the proper way to stretch can cause more harm than good. It is essential to set your expectations at the beginning so that you are aware of what it entails and know how to get the best results. That's what I want for you, I want you to get the best possible results, and that is only achievable through moving forward in the right way.

The Right Form

The proper form refers to the right execution of each and every stretch; this will make sure you will get the best out of your stretching routine. Many stretching exercises focus on isolated muscle groups, so when you are stretching, you will know where you should feel it. Paying attention to where you feel the stretch and how you are stretching, in general, is a vital part of getting a good workout.

Stretching causes tension in your muscles, so when you feel this, you know that you are working on something. However, it should never cause pain. If you do feel pain, then that is an indication that you are doing something wrong or have stretched too far for your muscles at this point. As soon as you feel pain, stop, assess why there was pain, and try and avoid that in the future. The saying "no pain, no gain" does not apply in this situation. Pushing yourself too far might result in torn muscles and damage to the tissues.

Make sure you have the right amount of space for the stretch. You do not want to be in mid-stretch and then be stopped by a piece of furniture or the wall. In most cases, you cannot modify a stretch for a smaller space, so if you try, you might not even get the benefits of that stretch. Make sure you know how to do the stretch before you attempt it. This will help you plan better both in terms of space and form. Knowing where your body is going with help with smoother transitions and a better experience overall.

Stretches are held for about 30 seconds or more; this is to make sure that your body has tension in the muscle. Doing it for too little time might not have as much of an effect as taking your time. Stretching is not about speed but rather about control, so focus on controlling your movements; this will make you more conscious about how you are executing your movements. Do not rush in and out of stretches; use your breathing as a guide if you need to. Slowing down your breathing can help you to slow down your movement and have more control.

A helpful tip is to watch yourself in the mirror. This way, you can see how you look when doing the stretch and pick up if you're doing something wrong much easier. Check your form in the mirror, especially with new and more difficult stretches. Once you are more comfortable, you can move away from the mirror. If you do not have a mirror, try recording yourself. It has the same effect, but you do not have to be confined to a room with a mirror.

Getting your form and execution right is one of the most important things you can do. It will prevent injury and make sure that you are getting the best out of your stretches. This will reduce frustration since many people feel like they aren't getting anywhere, but this is just because they are not doing the stretches correctly. Once you learn how to perform the stretches correctly, half the battle is won. It will make the whole experience better and more worthwhile.

It Takes Time

Like with many things in life, stretching is all about consistency and effort. You won't suddenly become flexible after one or two stretching sessions; it takes time. Think about it, your body has not been flexible for your whole life, and now you are going to have to retrain your muscles. It might take a few months to start getting your flexibility, but it is all worth it, and hard work will pay off in the end.

You should be stretching every day, but if you cannot commit to this, then try for three to four times a week. If you do not do it often enough, then you might lose the flexibility you have gained, consistency is key. The amount of time that you spend on stretching for each session can vary depending on a few factors, but the important thing is to have a plan and then stick to it. Ten minutes of stretching every day will have greater benefits than two hours of stretching every other week. Remember, we are training our muscles to behave in a certain way.

Make it a routine, write it down somewhere so that you do not forget. Once you make it a priority, you are more likely to do it, and the more you do it, the better it will be for you. It will definitely help to plan out your stretching routine before you do it, you are more likely to stick to something if it is planned out. Plan it out a week in advance, know what you are doing for the whole week; that way, you just have to jump into the routine. This will help with consistency. I know all this seems obvious and trivial, but this is because people seriously do overlook the simple things, planning a stretching routine before they do it or making sure to do it for the full amount of time.

It might be hard in the beginning, the first time doing anything is hard, but keep at it and don't get discouraged.

The results that await you on the other side is well worth the time and effort. Consistency always brings the greatest rewards.

MOBILITY AND FLEXIBILITY TEST

Mobility and flexibility go hand in hand, but they are not interchangeable, so it is crucial to work on both of them. Too much of one and not enough of the other could lead to injuries down the line. Bedosky (2018), shows us the difference between mobility and flexibility. Mobility deals with the joints and their range of movement, having excellent mobility means that you can move your joints through their full range of movement without any pain, discomfort, or restriction. Flexibility focuses on the lengthening of the muscles; good flexibility refers to being able to stretch and bend your muscles without restriction and tightness. Both of these take work to improve on, but they should be worked on together in order to get the best results.

We all need a place to start, and for us to start at the right place, we need actually to know what our current ability is. Elorreaga (2018) developed a mobility test that will help you determine where you are in terms of mobility and flexibility. This test is divided into sections depending on what part of the body is being focused on. Before you move forward in your journey, it is wise to do the test and see what you need to focus on more and why certain parts of your body are tight. I will take you through each assessment, which can all be done at home. This is not to replace any advice given by a doctor or physiotherapist; at the end of the day, I am not there with you, so if your qualified health professional has given you instruction or advice, then you should go with that. These assessments are designed to provide you with a benchmark for your mobility, but they do not diagnose any medical problems.

Our bodies will give us different results when it is warmed up and when our muscles are cold. Try and do these assessments once when your muscles are stiff, since that will give you an idea of your everyday mobility and flexibility. Then do it again when your muscles have warmed up, maybe after a workout so that you can compare.

You may be tempted to skip a few that you think you can easily do; I can assure you it's likely your mobility could shock you with how bad it is, so it is worth trying all moves to assess where your problem areas are.

UPPER BODY MOBILITY

The following movements will determine your mobility or flexibility in various upper body joints and muscles.

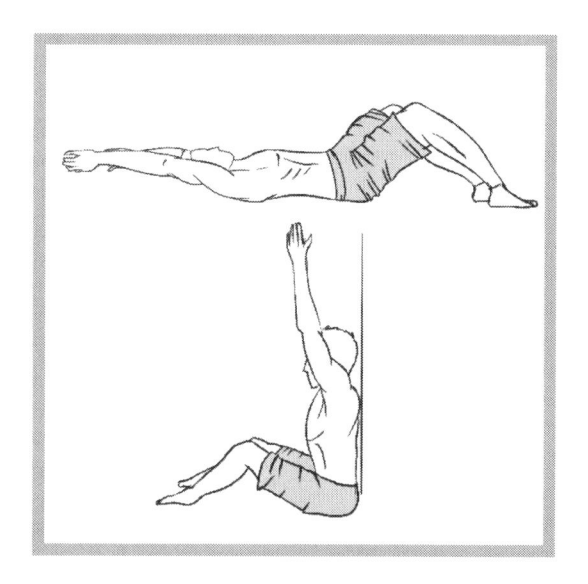

Shoulder Flexion

This move is designed to target your shoulder flexibility and mobility. It will show your ability to move your arms above your head at an increasing angle, away from your torso.

Flexibility Test Instructions:

- Lay on the ground, with the back flat.
- Raise your arms so that they move over your head.
- Your arms should lay flat on the ground behind you, without you having to arch your back.
- Your arms should not be bent, and your ribs should not be excessively flaring.

If you are unable to do this, then it indicates that you might have tight lats, pecs, biceps long head, rotator cuff, triceps, or a low thoracic extension. If you can do this, then you have excellent overhead flexibility.

Mobility Test Instructions:

- Sit with your back straight up against the wall.
- Same as the previous test, lift your arms so that they are above your head.
- They should be touching the wall without an arched back, bent arms, or flared rib cage.

If you are unable to do this and were able to do the previous test, then this indicates that you have low overhead mobility. You may suffer from weak or tight rotator cuffs, serratus anterior, or lower traps. If you were able to do this, then you have excellent overhead mobility.

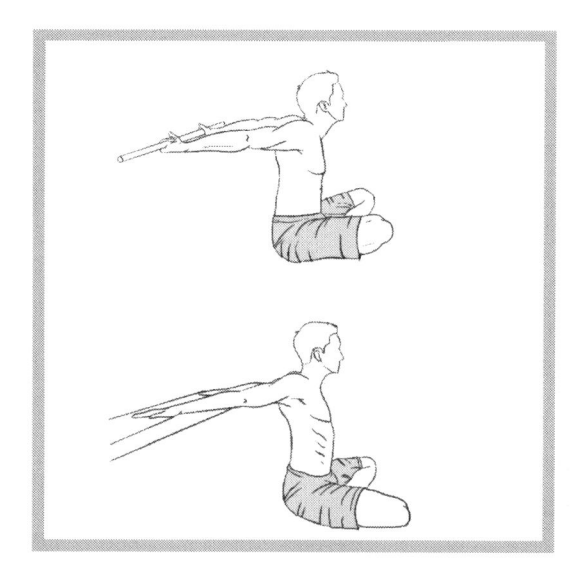

Shoulder Extension

These moves are designed to test your shoulder hyperextension.

Flexibility Test Instructions:

- Place your hands behind you, on a box or any other flat surface.
- Your palms should be flat against the surface.
- Crouch down.
- You should be able to get at least a 45-degree angle from your torso to your arm. 90 degrees if you are a gymnast or athlete, where that is needed.
- Your spine should not be rounding.

If you can do this, then you have between satisfactory and good shoulder extension flexibility. If you find this difficult, then you may have tight pecs, anterior delts, or biceps.

Mobility Test Instructions:

- Hold onto a broomstick or rod, with both hands behind you. Try this with your knuckles facing upwards (supine grip) and with your knuckles facing downward (prone grip).
- List the stick or rod upwards, with your elbows straight.
- You should get a 90-degree angle or more.

If you are unable to do this, then you may have weak rotator cuffs, posterior delts, or lats.

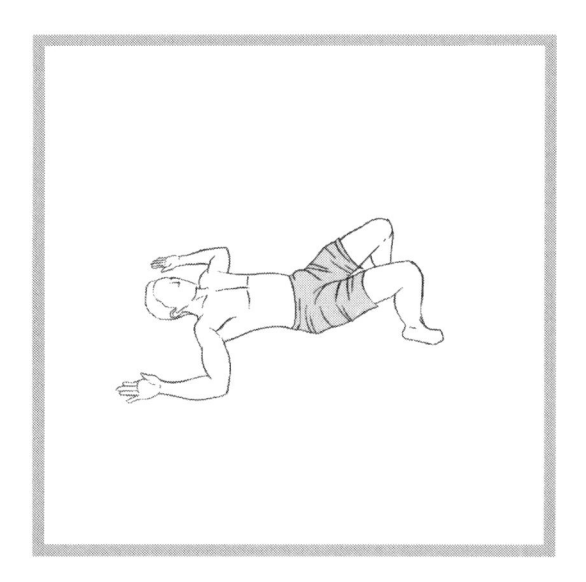

External Rotation

This move tests how well your shoulders rotate outwards.

Flexibility Test Instructions:

- Lay on the ground with your arm straight out beside you. There should be a straight line formed from your right hand all the way to your left hand.
- Bend your elbows upwards at a 90-degree angle.
- Your palms should be facing the ceiling, and the back of your hands should be flat against the floor.
- Your back should remain flat against the floor.

If you can have the backs of your hands and your back flat against the floor at the same time, then you have good external rotation. If not, then you may have tight internal rotators.

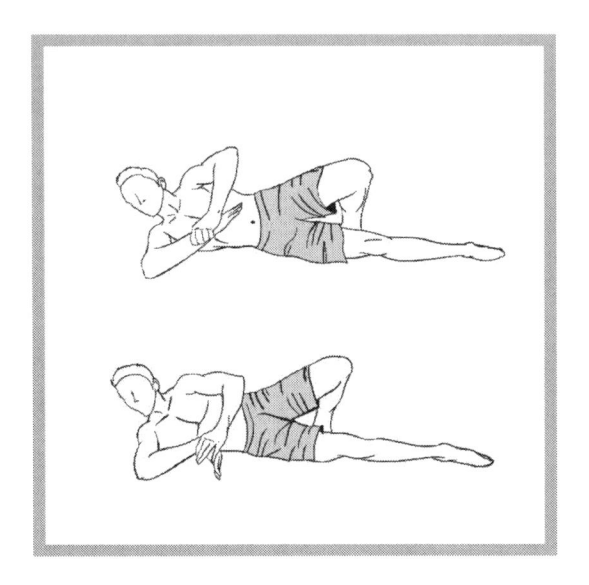

Internal Rotation

This move is designed to test how well your shoulders rotate inwards.

Flexibility Test Instructions:

- Lie down on your back. Move your body over to one side so that one side of your body is resting on the floor.

- Your arm should be about 70 degrees out from your body, with your fingers pointing to the sky.
- Pivot your arm so that your palm starts moving towards the floor, go as low as you can.
- Flex your wrist so that your fingertips touch the floor.

If you can do this, then you have good internal rotation flexibility. If you find this difficult, then it indicates that you may have tight external rotators or a tight posterior capsule.

Mobility Test Instructions:

- Place the back of your hand flat against the small of your back.
- Your scapula (shoulder blade) should be flat; it should not be sticking out.
- Move your hand up your back towards your head.
- Bring your other hand up and over your head towards the side, moving up your back.
- Try and grab the fingers of the hand, moving up the back without the scapula sticking out.

If you can do this, then your internal rotation mobility is good. If not, then you may have a weak teres major, subscapularis, serratus anterior, or lower traps.

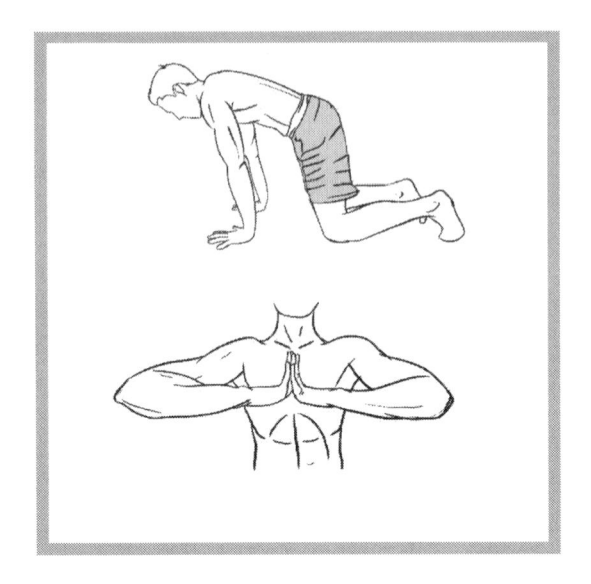

Wrist and Finger Extension

This move is designed at testing how well you can open up your wrists and fingers.

Wrist Flexibility Test Instructions:

- Get down on all fours, with your palms flat on the floor.
- Your hands should be aligned with your shoulders.
- Keep your hands straight and lean forward as far as you can.
- The palms of your hands should remain stuck to the floor at all times.

USE IT OR LOSE IT

If you can do this with your arms pushing past more than 90 degrees, then you have good wrist flexibility. If not, it indicates that you have tight wrists.

Finger Extension Test Instructions:

- Place your hands together, with palms and fingers touching.
- Slowly move the bottoms of your hands apart.
- Move as far apart as you can with the entirety of your hands still touching.

If you can do this and get a 90-degree angle from the back of your hand to your fingers, then you have good finger flexibility. If not, then you will have to work on it.

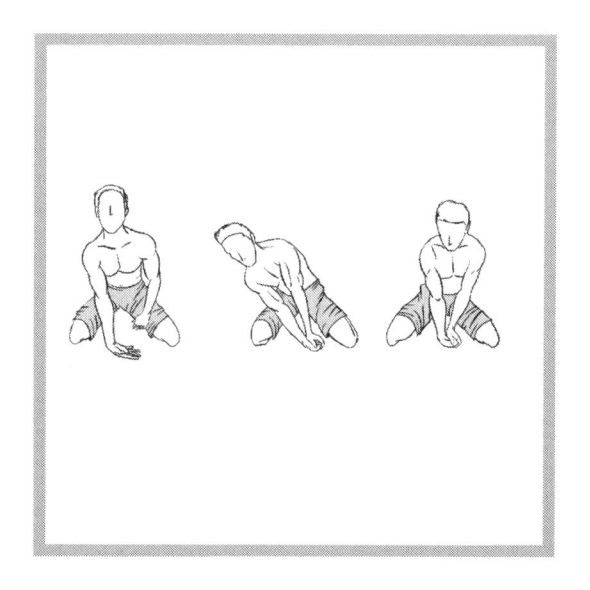

Wrist and Finger Flexion

This move tests how far your wrists and fingers move inwards.

Flexibility Test Instructions:

- Get down onto your knees, place the back of one of your hands on the floor, between your legs.
- Lean over to one side; this should be the side the arm is on. For example, if you are using your right arm, then lean over to the right.
- Roll your fingers up into a ball, so you are making a fist. The back of your hand remains on the ground.
- Slowly move your body back towards the center; your arm should stay straight.

If you can get back to the center with your arm perpendicular to the floor, then your wrist and finger flexion is at a good level. If not, then you will have to work on it.

LOWER BODY MOBILITY

The following movements and stretches will focus on the lower body and help you to identify any problem areas in that region.

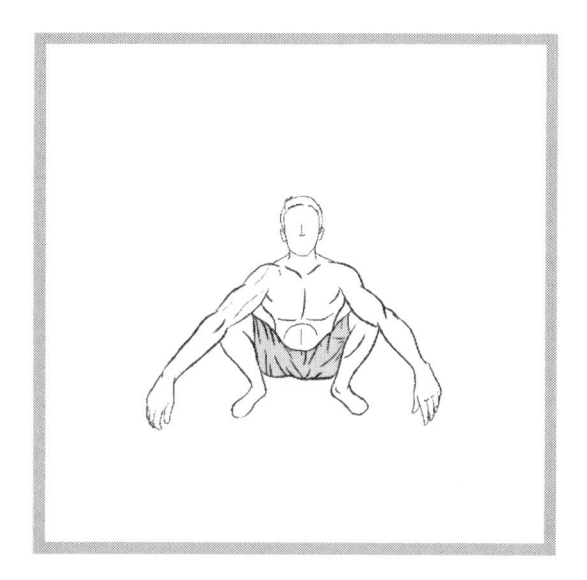

Internal Hip Rotation

This movement will test how well your hip moves inwardly. There aren't many situations where you would be doing this naturally, but it is good to have it balance out external hip rotations, which are more common.

Instructions:

- Start in a rested squat position. Go down as low as you can.
- Lean over to the right and drop the left knee in towards the floor.
- Your foot should not leave the floor. However, it is expected that it will shift over to the side.

- Touch your knee to the ground.
- Repeat on the other side.

If your knee can touch the ground, then you have good internal hip rotation.

For those that cannot get into a rested squat position, there is another move that you could try.

Instructions:

- Lay flat on your belly with your legs bent so that your legs are at a 90-degree angle.
- Let your feet drop to the sides of your body simultaneously.
- Your legs should make an angle of over 35 degrees.

If you can reach more than a 35-degree angle, then your internal hip rotation is satisfactory, but a 45-degree angle is preferable.

If you were unable to do both of these moves, then it indicates that you have tight external rotators or tight glutes.

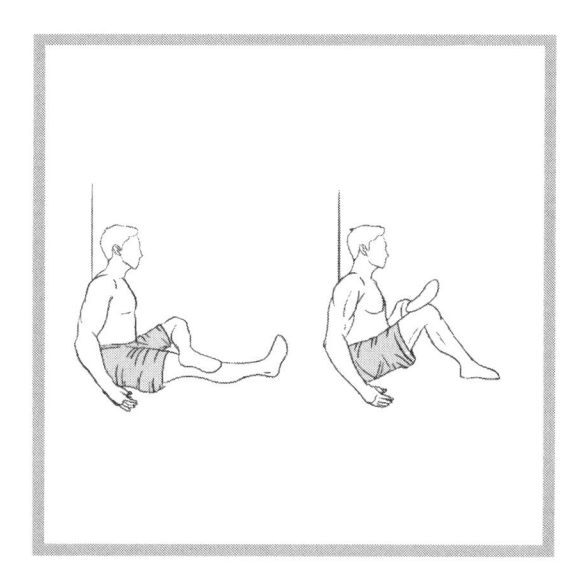

External Hip Rotation and Hip Flexion

This will test how well your hips can move and rotate outwardly.

Instructions:

- Sit up straight with your back flat against a wall.
- Stretch your legs out straight in front of you and bring your left leg over your right knee. Your left ankle should be touching the right knee.
- Bring your right knee up as high as you can go.
- You may repeat on the other side if desired, to see if you get different results.

If you can get your left leg (in this case) up to your chest, then you have really good flexibility. However, about 45 degrees away from your chest is satisfactory. If you are unable to get this close, then you probably have a tight TFL (tensor fascia lata; part of your hip muscles), piriformis, or glutes.

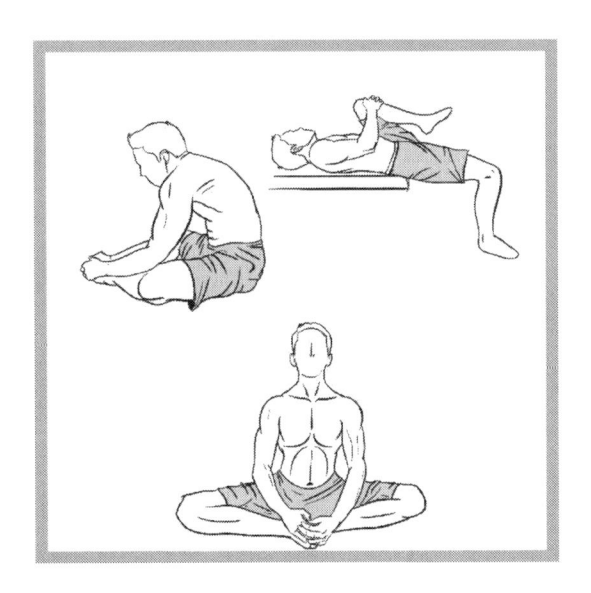

Hip Abduction and External Hip Rotation

This move will test how far your leg can move away from your midline, think of doing a side-kick or leg lift.

Instructions:

- Start by sitting on the floor on your sit bones; your back should be straight. Make sure you are not on your tailbone.
- Bring your feet together, so the bottoms are touching.
- Pull your feet into your body and try and push down your knees to touch the floor.

If your feet are brought in as much as they can go, and you can get your knees to touch the ground, you are pretty flexible. If not, then you probably have tight adductors and internal rotators.

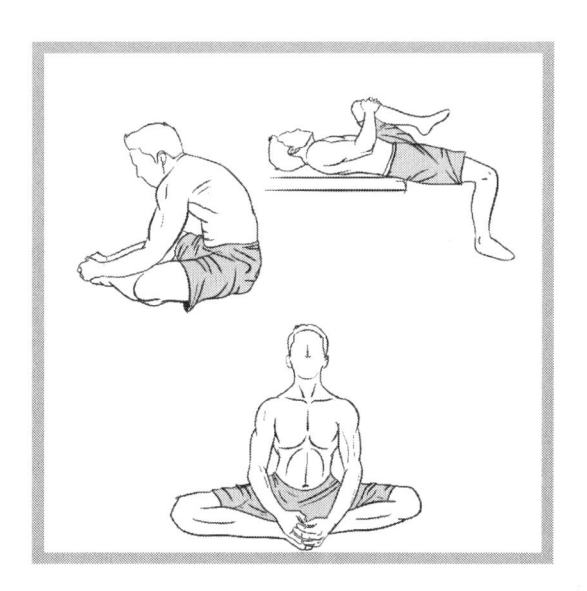

Hip Extension

A good hip extension will allow your leg to move behind you.

Instructions:

- Lie down on your back, on a hard flat surface. The best place would be a table or a bench.
- Your whole back should be on the surface with your butt half on and half off.
- Bring your right knee up to your chest, bring it in as close as you can and push your back into the surface.
- Allow your left leg to hang off the edge of the surface. Your knee should be bent at a 90-degree angle.
- Your leg should hang past the edge of the surface, at an angle over 180 degrees. Your back should never leave the surface.

If your leg hangs over the surface and is not pulled upwards, then you have a good hip extension. If you are unable to do this, then you probably have tight hip flexors or tight quads. If you notice that your leg moves outwards, then you probably have weak adductors or a tight TFL.

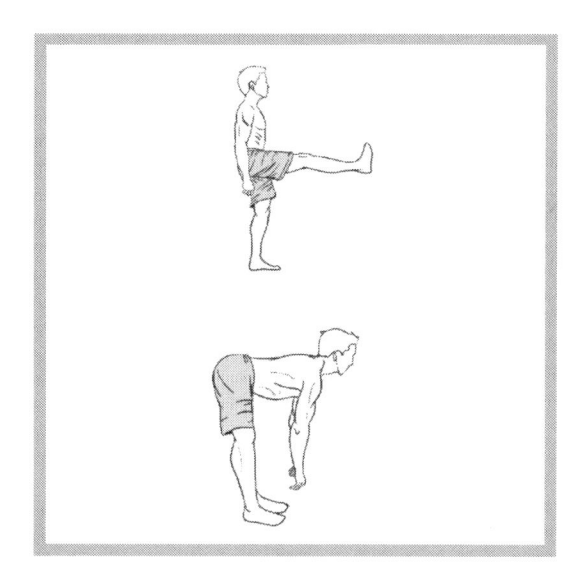

Pike

The pike position is just a forward bend, but you can feel it in the muscles of your leg.

Pike Flexibility Test Instructions:

- Start by standing up straight with your feet together.
- Bend over at your hips, keeping your back straight.
- Keep your knees locked.
- Try and get down as low as possible with your back still straight.

If you can get your back to lay 90 degrees from your legs, then you have satisfactory pike flexibility. For those more flexible, you can try and touch your palms to the ground about two feet from your legs. If you are unable to get a minimum of the 90-degree angle, this indicates that you have tight hamstrings, calves, and Achilles tendons.

Pike Mobility Test Instructions:

- Start by standing up straight.
- Kick one of your legs out in front of you without bending either knee or your back.
- Try and get your leg up to a 90-degree angle, right out in front of you.

If you are unable to get your leg up to 90 degrees, then this indicates that you may have weak hip flexors and a weak rectus femoris.

Ankle Dorsiflexion

This movement tests the mobility of your ankle. It is important to have strong ankles as they are part of what holds us up and helps us to keep moving.

Instructions:

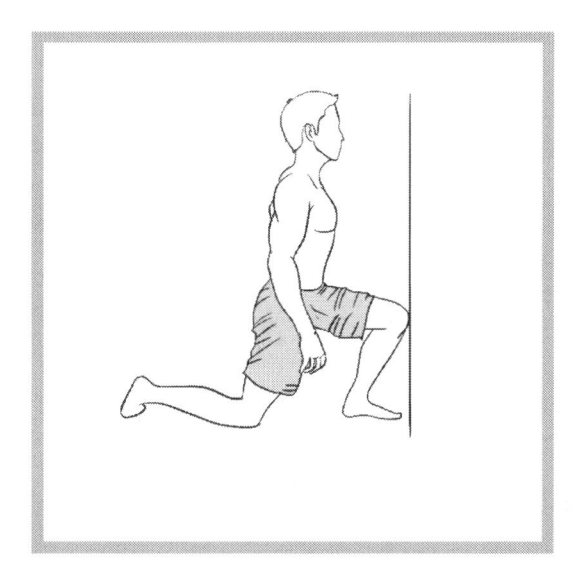

- Start by getting into a lunge position by a wall. Your knee and toe of one leg should be touching the wall, while the other leg is out behind you.
- Place a ruler underneath your foot or right beside it.
- Move your foot backward an inch at a time. Your knee should remain fixed to the wall.
- Once you have reached five inches, you may stop. Make sure the heel of your foot never lifts off the ground.

If you can reach the five inches away from the wall, this shows that your dorsiflexion is good. If not, then this is an indicator that you may have a tight soleus or Achilles tendon.

If you are finding yourself having a mobility or flexibility problem with a muscle you didn't even know existed, you do not need to worry. As long as you know, it is in your back or hip or wherever, that is okay. I am going to provide you with stretches to cover all areas that will certainly target that obscure muscle you haven't heard of and improve that problem area.

CONCLUDING THOUGHTS ON THE MOBILITY AND FLEXIBILITY TEST

Once you have completed the mobility and flexibility test, you should have a good idea of where your problem areas lie. I know this seems like a lot, but I am confident this will not take you long and will provide you with an excellent gauge of where you are right now. Do not feel discouraged if you are unable to do some or even all of the moves; that is why I wrote this book. I want to help you along your journey of regaining flexibility and mobility.

In order to move forward, you needed to know where you

are right now. Now that you are entirely aware of what you are capable of and what you need to improve on, we can begin giving you the tools you need to succeed at your goal of increased mobility and flexibility.

2

CONDITIONING: ALL THE STRETCHES YOU WILL EVER NEED TO KNOW

The stretches that are mentioned in this chapter will be focused on resolving short term problems. Sometimes we sit or sleep funny, and that causes our muscles and joints to hurt. I'm sure you have woken up with a stiff neck from sleeping in an uncomfortable position. This sort of thing is very common and doesn't usually have any long term damage, but it does cause discomfort. When you are uncomfortable or sore, you will not perform at your best. Stretches are the best way to get rid of that pain and discomfort so you can get back to feeling your best.

The stretches below are broken up into body part specific stretches. This will help you navigate the chapter easier, and if you have a specific problem, you know where to find the solution. Let's get into the stretches.

NECK, SHOULDER, AND CHEST

Many people suffer from some sort of tightness or discomfort in these areas. This is usually due to the way we sit at our computers or the way we sleep. Whatever the cause, it can be very uncomfortable to deal with. The following stretches will help relieve tension, stiffness, and discomfort from the chest, neck, and shoulders.

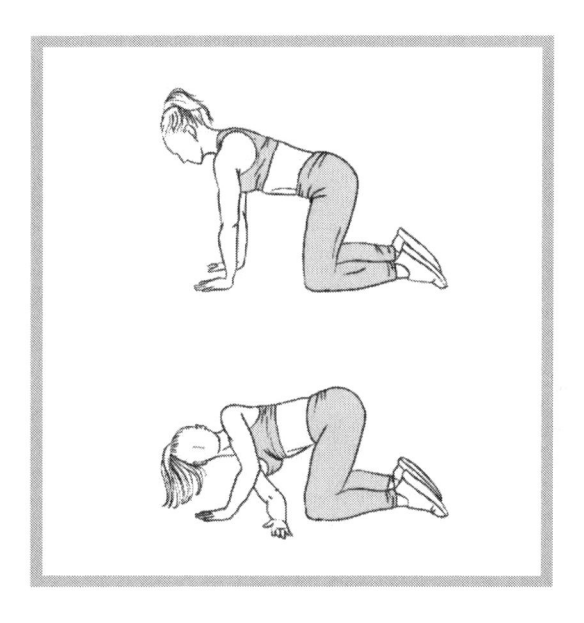

Thread the Needle

This stretch targets your shoulder girdle muscles and a muscle in your chest called the pectoralis minor.

Instructions:

- Begin by kneeling down on all fours; your hands should be aligned with your shoulders and your knees with your hips.
- Take your right arm and stretch it through the space between your left arm and thigh. Your palm should be facing up.
- Bend your left arm to allow the right side of your body to have more movement. You should be able to feel it at the back of the right shoulder.
- Hold for a couple of seconds, repeat a few more times before moving on to the other side.

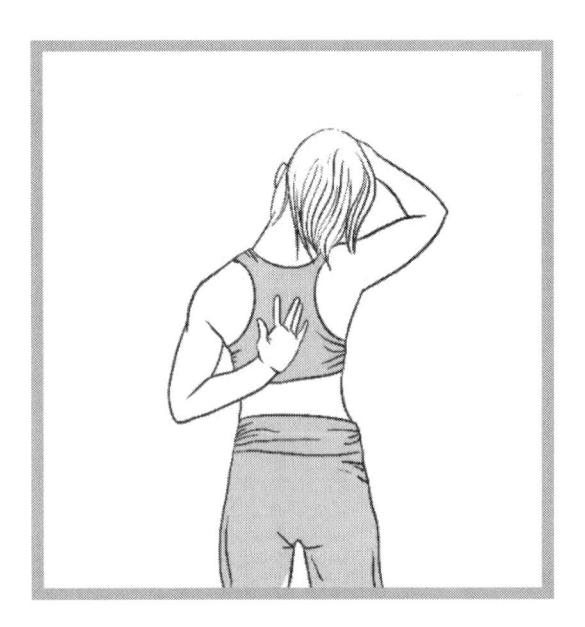

Upper Trapezius Stretch

This stretch will target your neck muscles; it gives the muscles a nice long stretch.

Instructions:

- Begin by sitting or standing with your back straight.
- Place one hand on your back; it can be on your lower back or between your shoulder blades.
- Take the other hand, place it to the opposite side of your head and pull your head to your shoulder.
- You should feel a stretch in your neck on the opposite side of the arm, pulling your head down. Hold for 20 to 30 seconds and then repeat on the other side.

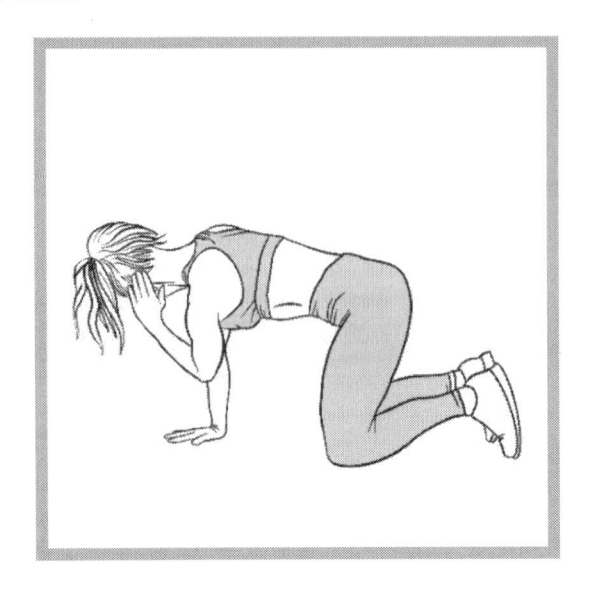

Quadruped Thoracic Rotation Stretch

This stretch targets the upper part of your spine.

Instructions:

- Begin on all fours. Align your hands with your shoulders and your knees with your hips. Your core should be engaged, and your back should remain straight at all times.
- Touch the back of your head with your right hand, do not put pressure on your head.
- Slowly move your head and shoulder inward towards your opposite arm.
- Then move all the way back, past the starting point

until your elbow points up to the ceiling.
- Return to the middle position after holding for a couple of seconds.
- Do this for about 30 seconds then repeat on the other side.

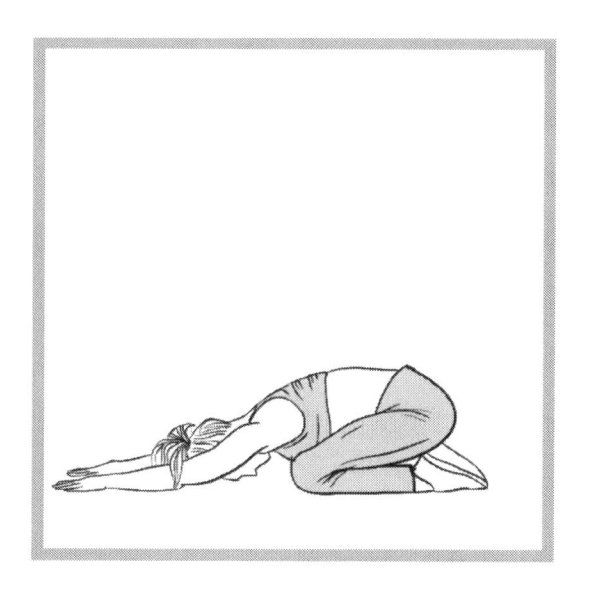

Child's Pose

This is a simple yoga move that helps with your neck, back, and shoulders. You should also feel it in your glutes and hips.

Instructions:

- Kneel on the floor and sit on your heels. Your knees

should be a bit wider than your hips, and your feet should be touching.
- Fold your body over so that your torso is lying on your thighs. Reach your arms out in front of you so that they are over your head. Place your forehead on the ground.
- Pull your chest and shoulders towards the floor; this will cause a deeper stretch.
- Hold this position for 30 seconds before repeating.

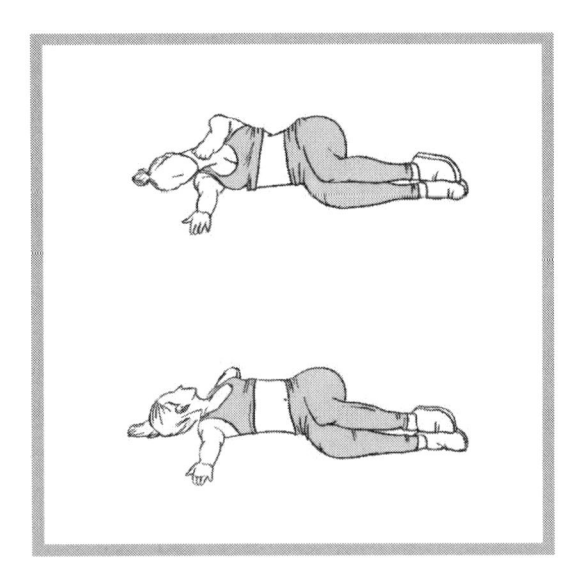

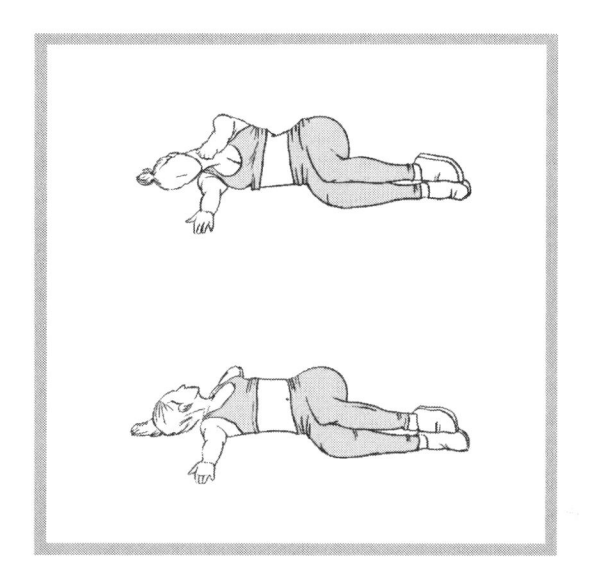

T-spine Windmill Stretch

This stretch targets many muscles in your shoulder.

Instructions:

- Lie down on your side with your arms stretched out in front of you, your knees and hips bent at a 90-degree angle.
- Lay your arms on top of each other and the same with your legs.
- Move your top hand over to the other side of your body; you should now be laying with both arms stretched out on opposite sides to form a T shape.
- Slowly return to the starting position.

- Repeat about 5 to 10 times before repeating on the other side.

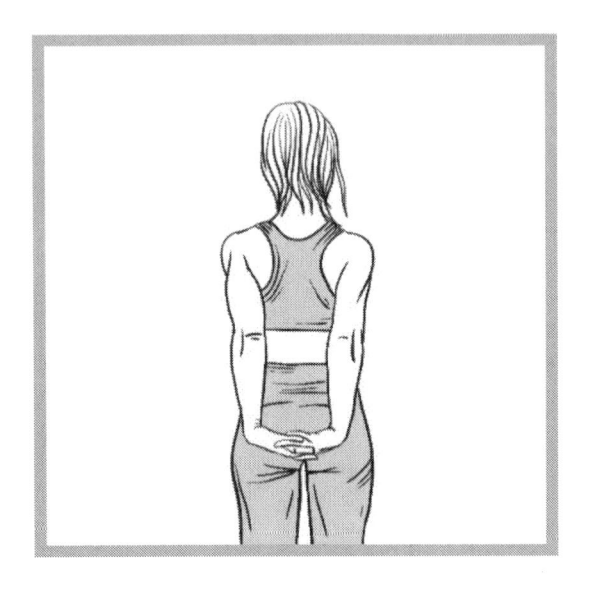

Reverse Shoulder Stretch

This stretch will target your deltoids and the pecs.

Instructions:

- Start by interlocking your fingers behind your back with your palms facing up.
- Your back and arms should be straight, and you should be pulling your shoulder blades together.
- Push your arms upward so that you can feel a stretch in your pec muscles.

- Hold this pose for about 30 seconds.

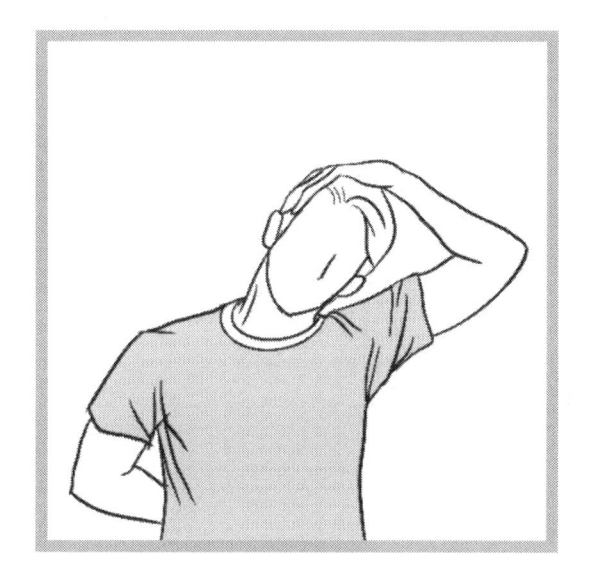

Cervical Side Bend

This stretch will help relieve the tension in the neck muscles.

Instructions:

- Sit or Stand with your back and neck straight.
- Move your right ear to your right shoulder, while you keep looking straight in front of you.
- You should feel the stretch in your left neck muscles. Hold for a few seconds and then repeat on the other side.

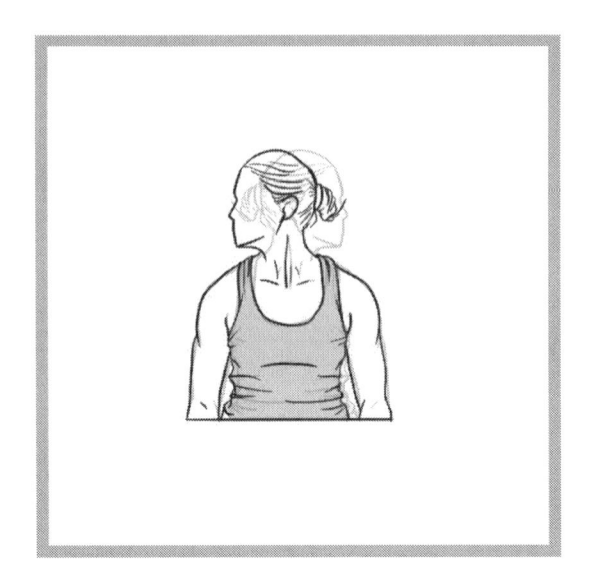

Cervical Rotation

This stretch also focuses specifically on the neck muscles.

Instructions:

- Turn your head to one side; make sure not to move your shoulders.
- Hold for a few seconds then turn to the other side.
- If you would like to add some pressure use your hand push against your chin gently.

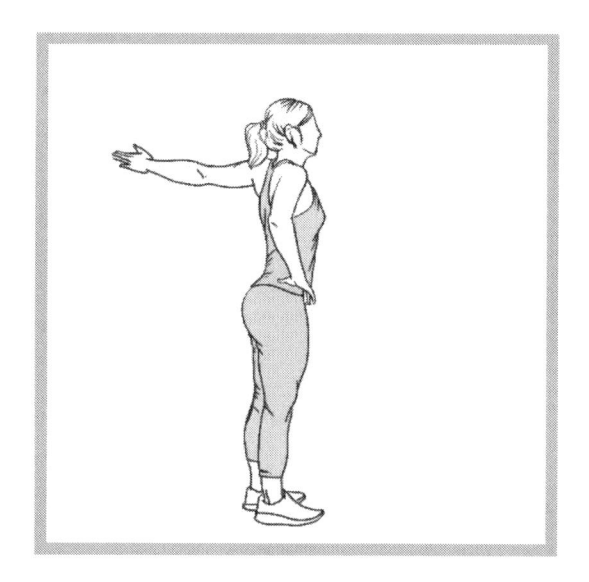

Wall Chest Stretch

This movement will allow you to stretch out your chest muscles.

Instructions:

- Place a straight arm on a wall.
- Take a step forward with the leg furthest away from the wall.
- Gently move your chest forward and feel the stretch in your chest.
- You may move your hand lower or higher on the wall to stretch out the various sections in your chest.

- Repeat the process on the other side

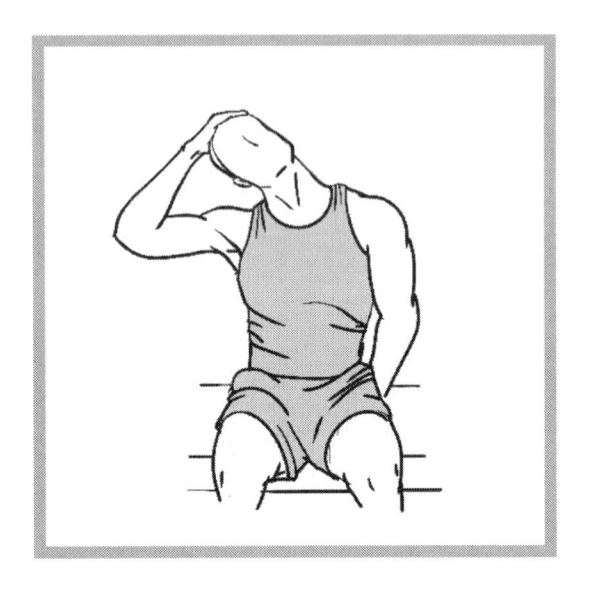

Anterior Scalene Stretch

Sometimes neck stiffness is caused by the anterior scalene muscle; this stretch will target that muscle.

Instructions:

- Place your right hand on your head.
- Start slowly pulling your head to the side so that your right ear moves closer to your right shoulder.
- Hold this pose for about 30 seconds and repeat three times before moving on to the other side.

ARMS, HANDS, AND WRISTS

When it comes to stretching, we often forget about our wrists, hands, and arms. However, these are important parts of our body and should not be neglected. If you are someone who is typing for most of the day, having any kind of discomfort or stiffness in these areas can really slow you down. There are a few stretches that can ease that feeling and help you get your mobility back.

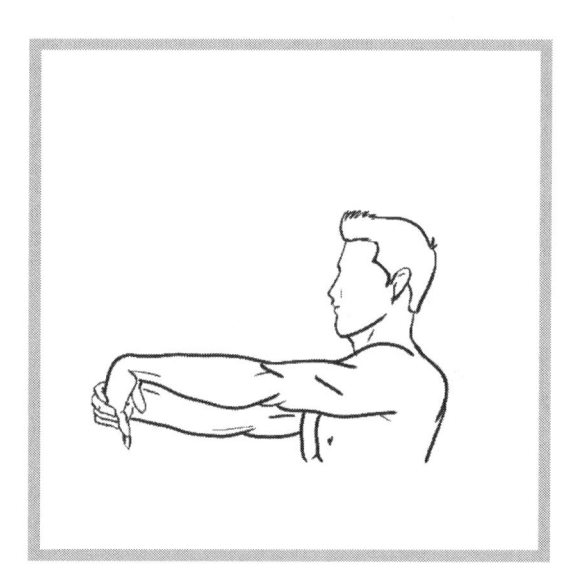

Wrist Extensor Stretch

This is a popular stretch to relieve tightness in your wrists.

Instructions:

- Lift your hand out in front of you and bend your wrist down so your palm faces you.
- Use your other hand to pull your bent wrist further towards you gently. You should feel the stretch in your forearm and wrist.
- Hold for 30 seconds and repeat three times. Repeat on the other hand.

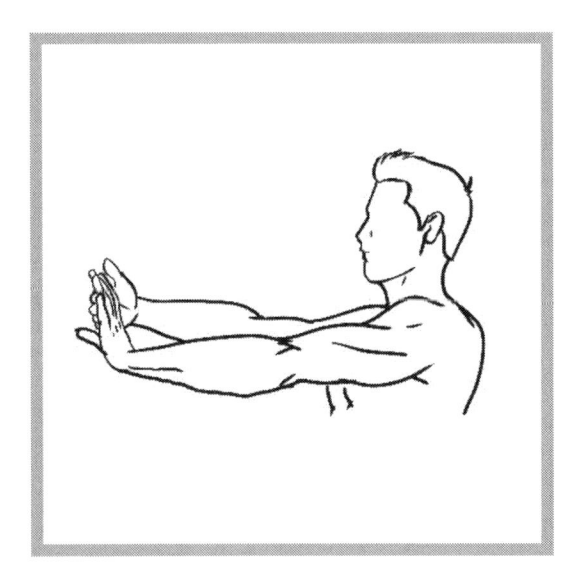

Wrist Flexor Stretch

This stretch is just the opposite of the previous stretch. It stretches the muscles on the inside of your wrist and arm.

Instructions:

- Stretch your hand out in front of you with your palm facing down.
- Bend your wrist upwards.
- Take the other and gently pull your wrist back towards you until you feel the stretch down your forearm.
- Hold for 30 seconds and repeat three times. Repeat on the other hand.

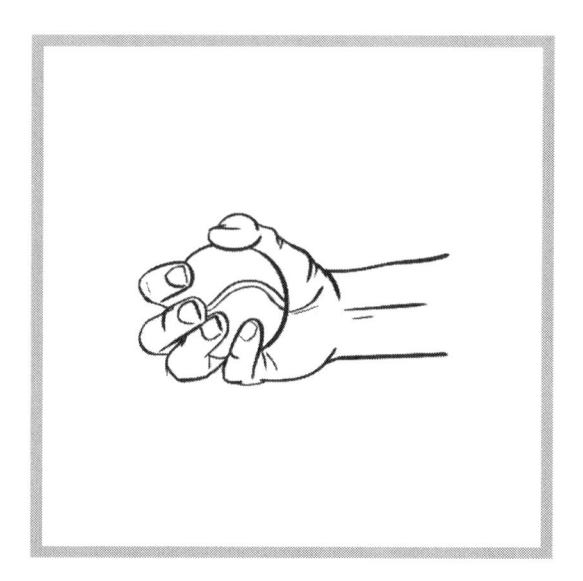

Tennis Ball Squeeze

This stretch targets the muscles and joints in the hand and wrist.

Instructions:

- Hold a tennis ball in one hand and squeeze it as hard as you can.
- Hold this for about 4 or 5 seconds then slowly release.
- Repeat this fifteen times before moving onto the other hand

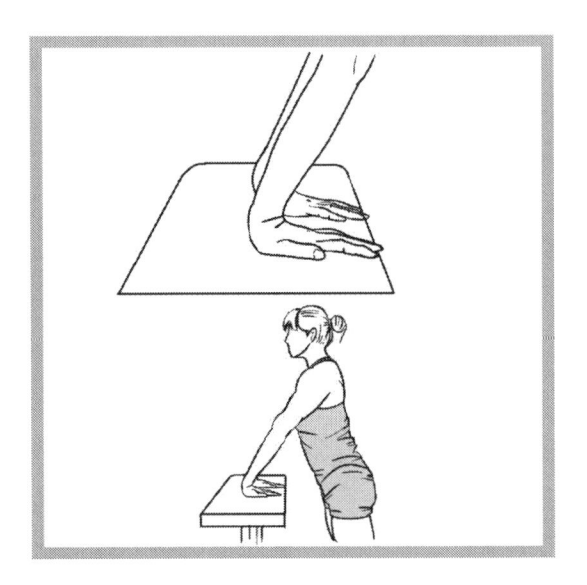

Desk Press

This stretch targets your wrists and forearms.

Instructions:

- Find a desk or table, place your hands on the

surface with your wrists turned, so your fingers are pointing at you.

- Gently push forward until you feel the stretch in your forearm.
- Hold for 15 seconds, repeat this about ten times.

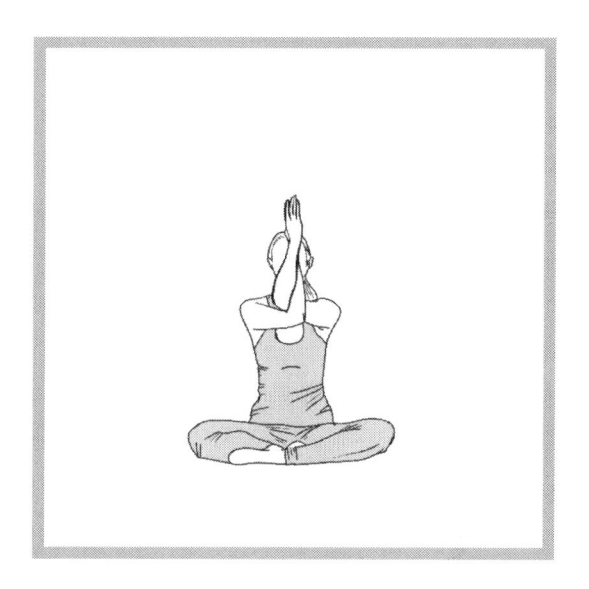

Eagle Arms

This stretch is excellent for stretching out your wrists and shoulders.

Instructions:

- Sit or stand up straight with your arms in front of you.

- Cross your left and right arms, with the right arm on top.
- Move both elbows, so they are bent upwards.
- Intertwine your arms so that the palms of both hands are touching.
- Move both arms away from your body in an upward motion; you should feel a spread between your shoulder blades.
- Stay in this pose for five deep breaths, then switch hands.

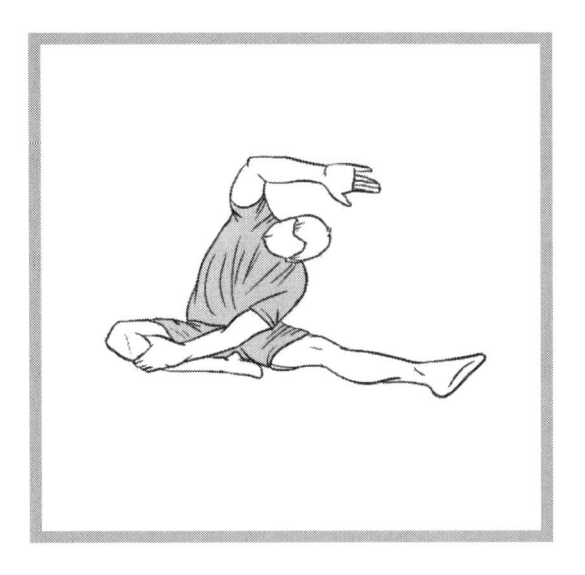

Assisted Side Bend

This move stretches out your arms but also lengthens your torso.

Instructions:

- Sit with your back straight.
- Move your arms so that they are above your head.
- Grab the wrist of one hand with the other and pull yourself over to the side.
- If you feel your ribs flaring, shift them back so that the stretch is only felt through your side and arm.
- Hold this for 30 seconds or until you feel ready, then switch over to the other side.

BACK AND TORSO

Suffering from a tight back can restrict your range of movement. The following stretches will allow you to gain back the mobility in your back.

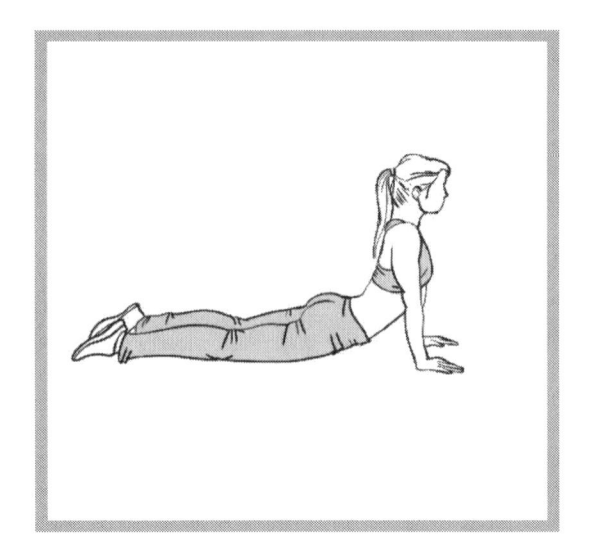

The Cobra

This stretch lengthens the whole upper body and is ideal if you suffer from pain related to sitting uncomfortably at a desk.

Instructions:

- Lay down with your belly to the floor.
- Bring your hands directly under your shoulders, breathe in and push up with your hands.
- Once your arms are completely straight, look up to the ceiling to stretch out your neck. Hold for about 30 seconds.
- Slowly exhale and bring yourself back down.

- Repeat this about three times.

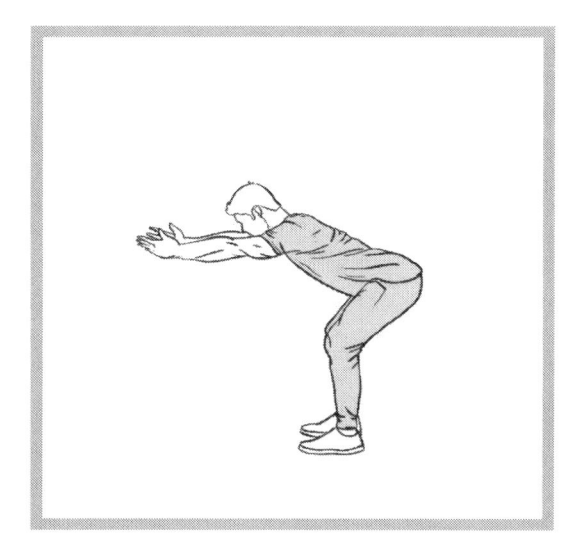

Hip Hinge

This stretch is especially useful for your lower back.

Instructions:

- Stand up with your back straight and your feet apart. You should be a few feet away from the wall.
- Leave your hands hanging to your side or out in front of you. Then bend your knees slightly, and bend at your pelvis, so your whole torso moves towards the ground.

- Once your back is parallel to the ground, slowly bring yourself back up to the starting position.

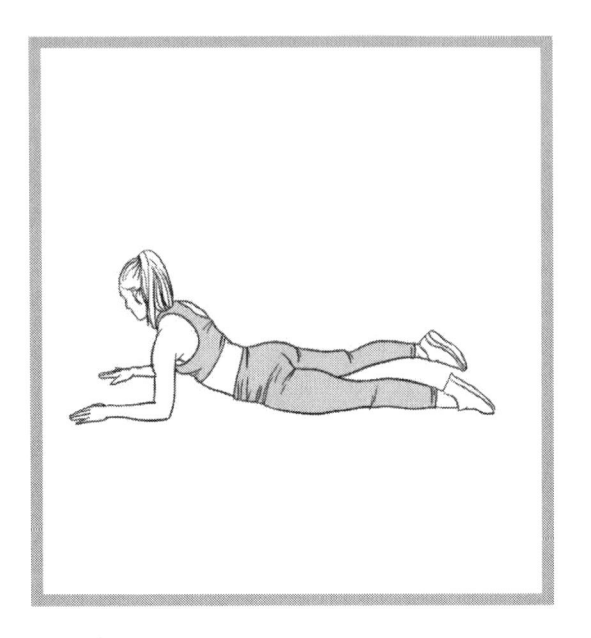

Sphinx Pose

This pose is common in yoga and is used to strengthen the spine and stretch out the abdomen.

Instructions:

- Begin by laying on your belly, the tops of your feet should be facing down.
- Bring your arms in and lift yourself up so your elbows and shoulders are in line. Your palms should

be flat on the ground, and your forearms should be parallel to each other.
- Inhale and push down on your forearms and lift your head and chest towards the ceiling.
- Engage your core and glutes, push your pelvis into the ground.
- Hold this pose for ten breaths and then relax and bring yourself back down slowly.

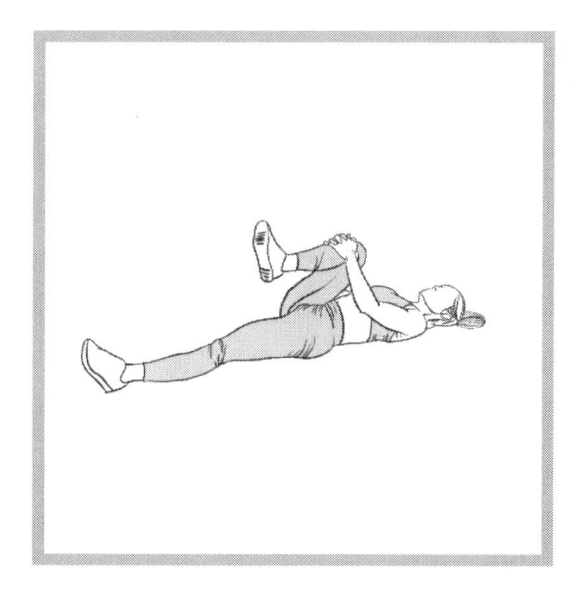

Knee-to-chest stretch

This stretch really targets the lower back.

Instructions:

- Lay flat on your back and bring your right knee up to your chest.
- With both hands, grab the shin of your right leg and pull it down so that you drive the leg into your chest. If this is too tricky, bend your left leg.
- Do not lift your hips, really try and lengthen your spine.
- Hold this pose for 5 to 30 seconds, release and then repeat at least three times before moving to the other leg.

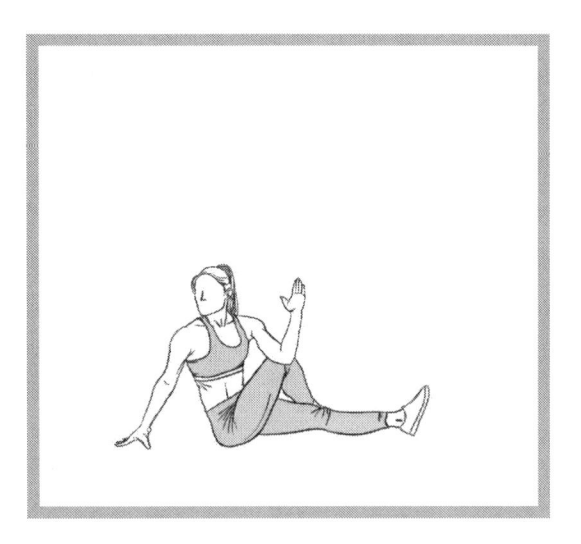

Piriformis stretch

This stretch will help release any tension in your buttocks, lower back, and hips.

Instructions:

- Lay down on your back and have your knees bent.
- Take your right ankle and place it over your left thigh.
- Grab your left thigh and pull it towards your chest, get as close to your chest as you can.
- Hold this pose for 30 to 60 seconds, then repeat on the other leg.

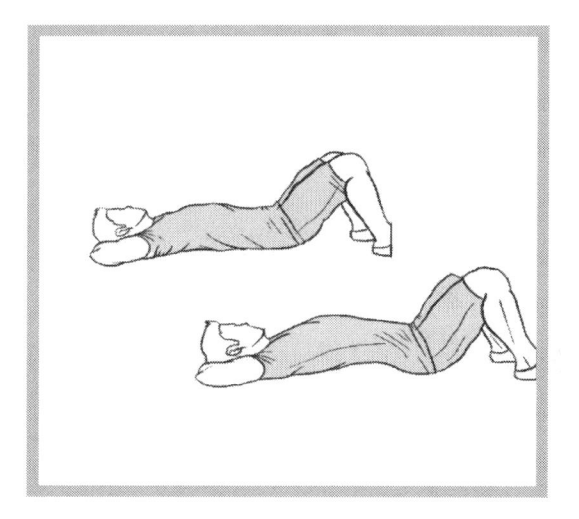

Pelvic tilt

This stretch can relieve pain and stiffness in your lower back and strengthen your abdomen.

Instructions:

- Lay on your back on the floor and your knees bent. Your hands should be to your side with palms flat on the floor.
- Flatten your back to the floor and engage your core muscles.
- Hold for 5 to 10 seconds and then slowly release. Repeat as many times as desired.

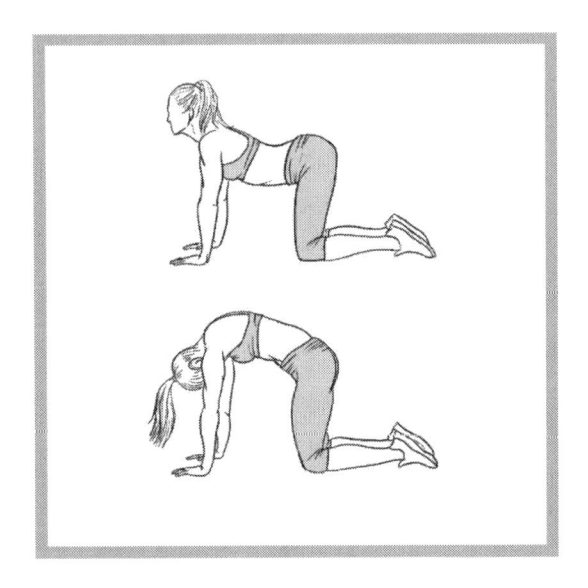

Cat-cow stretch

This move stretches out your spine and your upper body.

Instructions:

- Start on all fours.

- Breathe in, push your belly towards the ground, and lift your head.
- Then in one smooth movement exhale, tuck your chin in and lift your spine to the ceiling.
- Do this repeatedly for about 60 seconds.

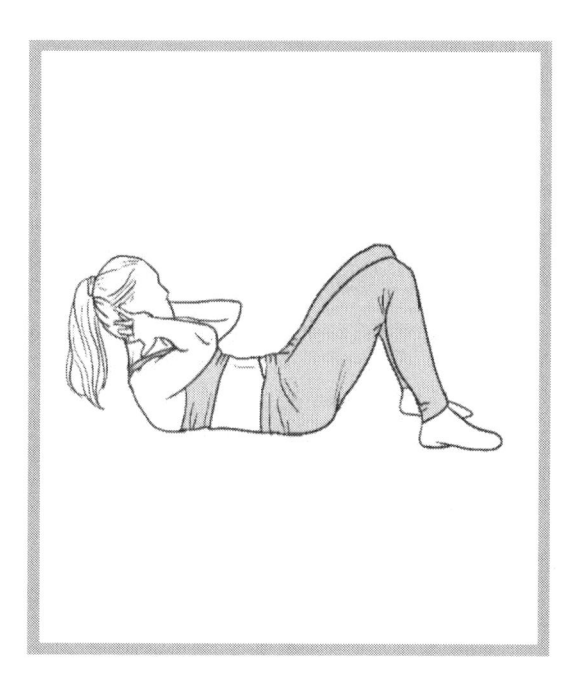

Partial Crunch

This move can stabilize your spine if you suffer or are recovering from back pain.

Instructions:

- Lay down on your back with your knees bent and feet on the floor.
- Push your lower back into the floor and engage your core.
- Lift your head and shoulders slightly off the ground by reaching for your feet with your hands. Use your core muscles, not your neck, to support this movement.
- Hold this for 1 to 3 minutes. Then relax and repeat.

HIPS AND GLUTES

Tight hips are something many people struggle with; sometimes, you will feel it when you sit. Your glutes are the biggest muscle in your body, so it is essential to pay attention to it, both of these areas work together when it comes to mobility and flexibility.

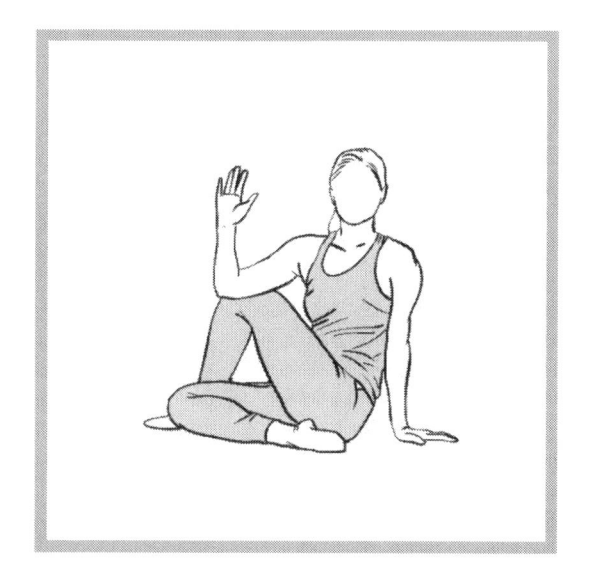

Half Lord of the Fishes

This stretch targets your spine and hips.

Instructions:

- Start by sitting on the floor, swing your left foot over your right thigh. Bend your right leg so your foot is as close to your butt as you can get it.
- Place your right elbow on the outside of your left knee and place your left hand just behind you for support.
- Keep your left foot firmly on the ground as you stretch.

- Hold for at least 30 seconds then repeat on the other side.

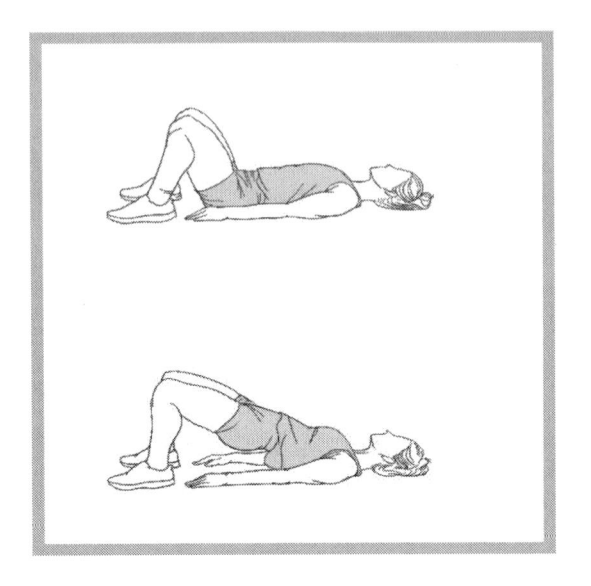

Glute Bridge

This exercise activates the glutes and works via a hip extension.

Instructions:

- Lay on your back, with your knees bent and feet hip-width apart.
- Lift your pelvis towards the ceiling by engaging your glutes and driving your heels into the ground.

- Hold for 5 to 10 seconds, then slowly bring yourself back down again. Repeat ten to fifteen times.

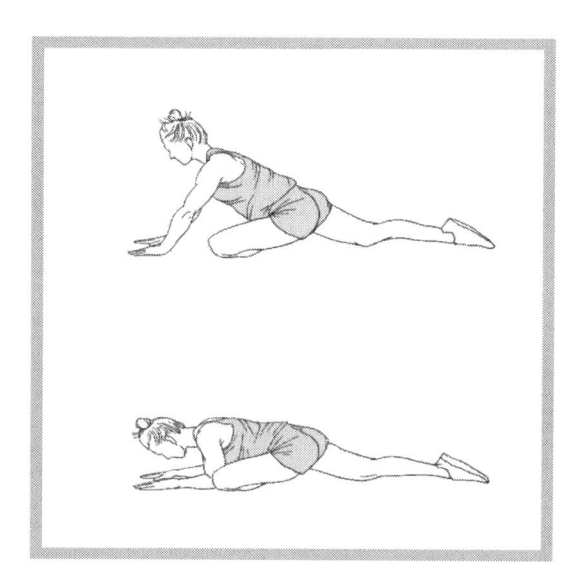

Pigeon Pose

This is an excellent stretch for those on their feet a lot as it stretches the glutes, hips, and piriformis.

Instructions:

- Start by getting down on your right knee. Drop your left knee to the left and slide your right leg behind you.
- Push your hips into the ground and walk your

hands forward on the ground as far as you can. Palms should be facing the ground.
- Keep your hips centered.
- Hold this pose for 20 to 30 seconds. Repeat on the other side.

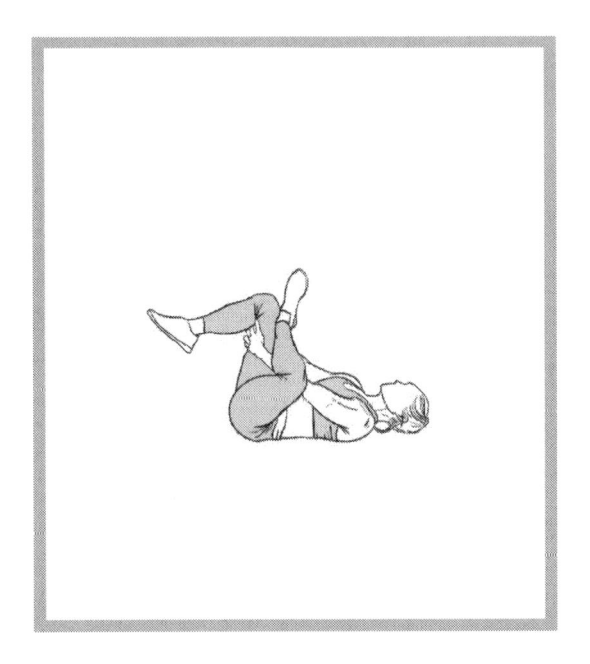

Lying Figure 4 Stretch

This move gives a great stretch to your glutes and hip flexors.

Instructions:

- Lay down on your back with your legs bent and feet off the ground.
- Place your right ankle over your left thigh.
- Grab your left thigh and pull both legs toward your chest.
- Hold for at least 20 seconds. Repeat on the other side.

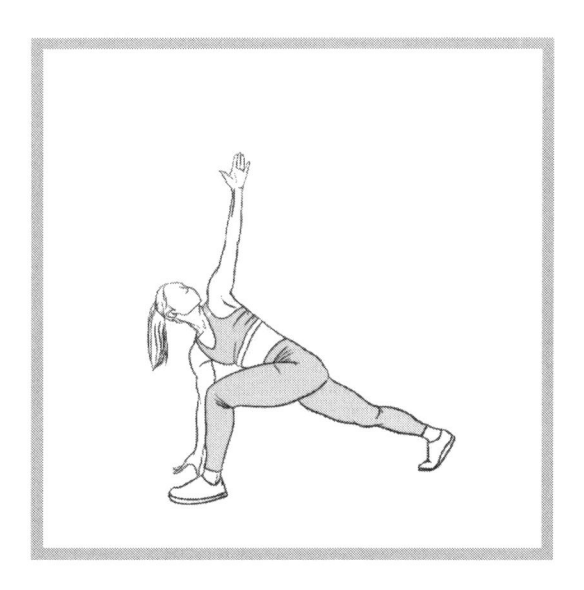

Lunge with Spinal Twist

This move will stretch out the hip flexors, back, and quads

Instructions:

- Stand up straight with your feet together, then take a large step forward with your right leg.
- Then drop your right knee, so you are in a lunge position. The back leg should be stretched out behind you.
- Put your left hand on the floor for stability and reach up to the ceiling with your right hand; this should cause your upper body to twist. Look up at your right hand.
- Hold for at least 30 seconds. Repeat with the left side.

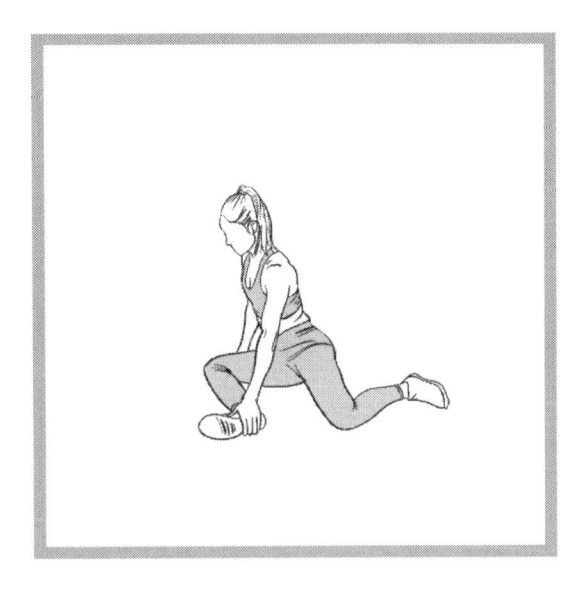

90/90 Stretch

USE IT OR LOSE IT

This stretch is designed to stretch out the tightness in the hips.

Instructions:

- Sit on the floor with your left leg out in front of you, bend it at a 90-degree angle. It should be flat on the ground with your foot flexed and facing the right.
- Move your right knee to the left of you and bend your knee and flex the foot; it should be facing behind you.
- Your left butt cheek should be on the ground, now try and get your right butt cheek as close to the ground as possible by pushing your hips downwards.
- Hold for at least 30 seconds and repeat on the other side.

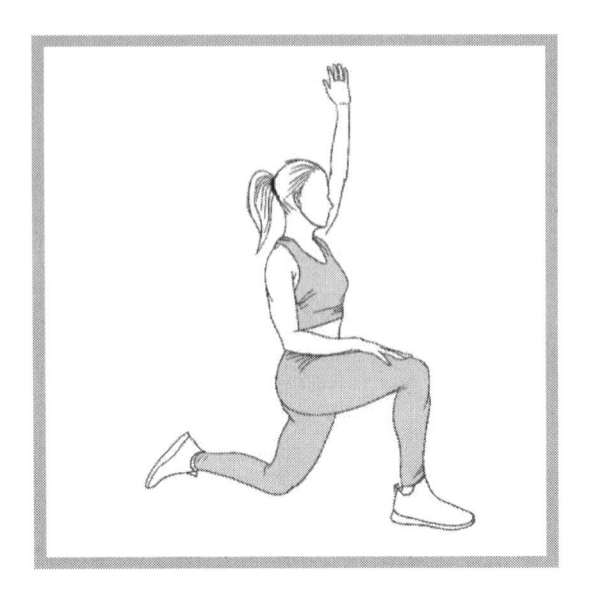

Lunging Hip Flexor Stretch

This stretch opens up the hips.

Instructions:

- Get down on one knee. One foot should be in front of you at a 90-degree angle, and the other should be bent behind you, the top of the foot flat on the ground.
- Lean forward as you try and push your hips towards the floor.
- Squeeze your butt and lift the arm on the opposite side of your front leg.

- Hold for 30 seconds and then repeat on the other side.

Knees and Thighs

Knee pain can really get in the way of our everyday lives. If there is tightness in our thighs, that might also contribute to pain in the knees. The following stretches will help with discomfort in your knee and thigh areas.

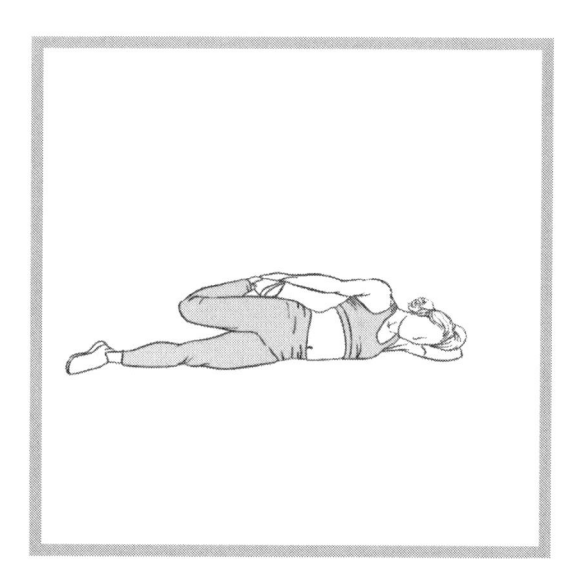

Quad Stretch

This stretch is designed to ease tension in the quads that might also be felt in the knee area.

Instructions:

- Lay down on your side with your legs stacked on top of each other. Use the arm closest to the ground to hold you up.
- Bend your top leg at the knee and grab your foot with your free hand.
- Pull the foot towards your butt until you feel the stretch in your quad.
- Hold this position for at least 30 seconds then repeat on the other side.

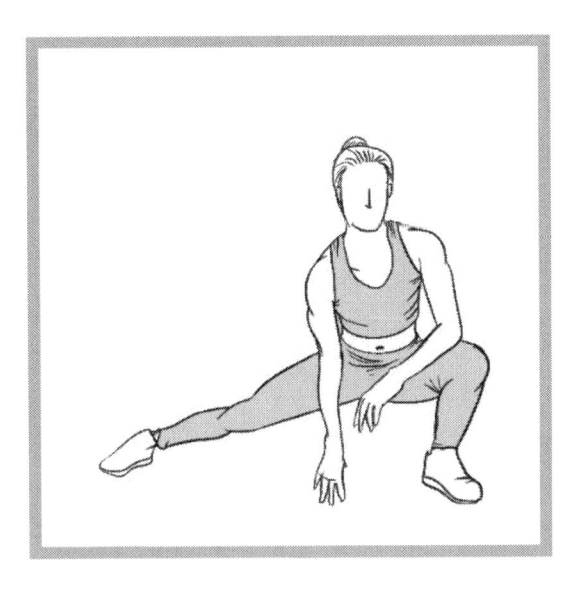

Side Lunge

This stretch targets your adductors (inner thigh muscles).

Instructions:

- Get into the side lunge position by stretching out one of your legs to the side and bending the other knee.
- Keep as much of the foot of the stretched leg on the floor as you can.
- You may place your fingertips on the ground if you need extra stability.
- Get as low as you can and hold for 15 to 30 seconds then repeat on the other side.

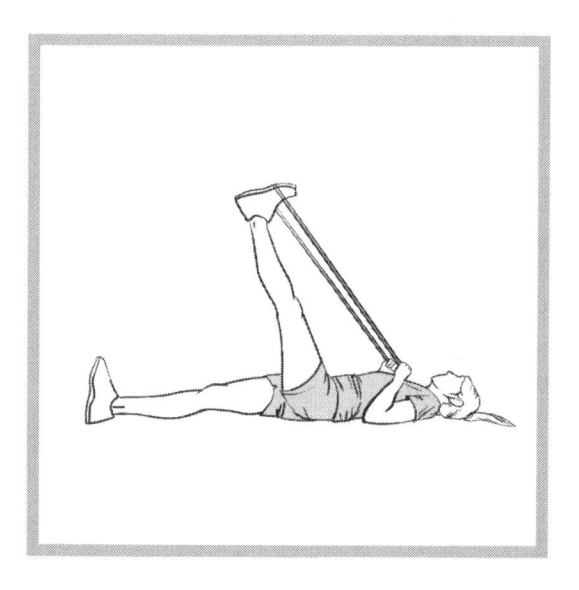

Supine Hamstring Stretch

This stretch is especially good for your hamstrings in your thighs.

Instructions:

- Lie down on your back with your knees bent.
- Use a towel or resistance bands to wrap around on your thigh and pull it towards you. The other leg can be bent, or you can straighten it out for more of a stretch.
- Try and keep the leg that you are pulling as straight as possible.
- Hold it as close to your body as possible for 30 to 60 seconds. Repeat three times, then switch to the other side.

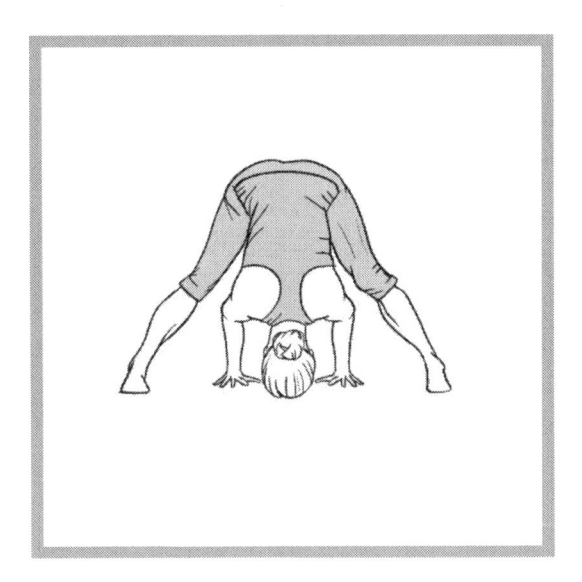

Wide-Legged Forward Fold

This stretch will target those thigh muscles.

Instructions:

- Stand with your legs 3 to 4 feet apart, could be wider depending on your height.
- Stand up straight and plant your feet into the ground, your feet should be parallel not facing inward.
- Breathe in, and as you exhale, bend at the hips, keeping your back nice and straight.
- Try and reach for the ground with your fingers, getting your head as close to the ground as possible.
- Hold this position for at least five breaths.

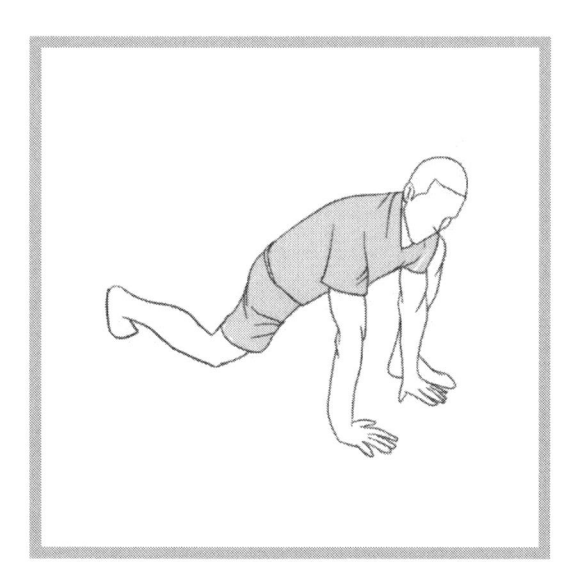

The Knight Stretch

This stretch is designed to stretch out your thighs and open up your hips.

Instructions:

- Get into the lunge position, with one leg bent down behind you and one bent up in front of you.
- Breathe in, push your chest outwards, and lean forward with your hips. Stretch it out as far as you can.
- Hold for 30 seconds and repeat five times on each side.

LOWER LEG, ANKLES, AND FEET

These parts of our body are the base of your body, and they need to be strong. Tight ankles can cause pain when walking, so it is important to get mobility back in these areas.

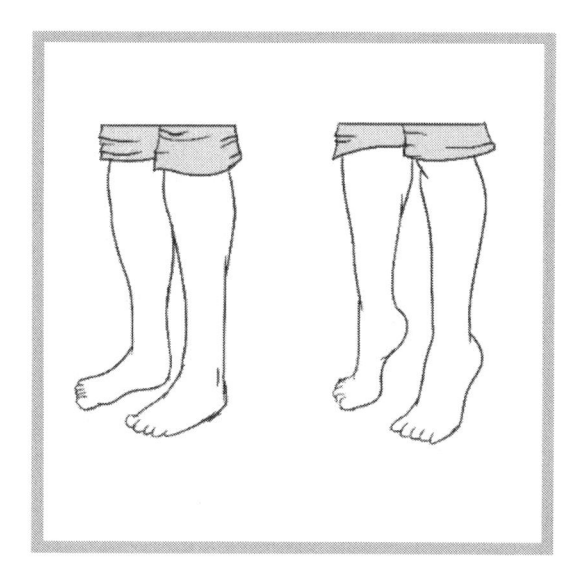

Tip Toe Tense

This stretch will stretch out the whole lower leg area.

Instructions:

- Stand up straight, then lift yourself onto your tiptoes.
- Hold for about 5 seconds, then bring yourself back down slowly and controlled.
- Repeat about ten to fifteen times.

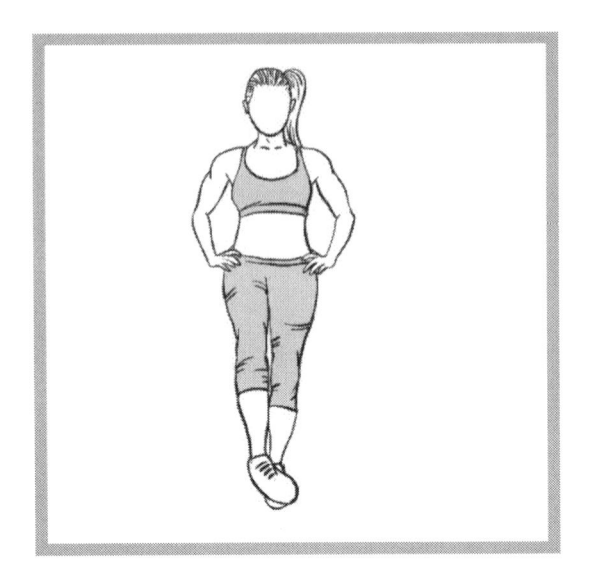

Ankle Rotation

This move will help with ankle stiffness.

Instructions:

- You may be lying down or sitting for this move.
- Lift your foot off the ground and rotate your ankle to the left, hold for a few seconds.
- Then rotate your ankle to the right, hold for a few seconds.
- You may do this as many times as desired. Repeat on the other foot.

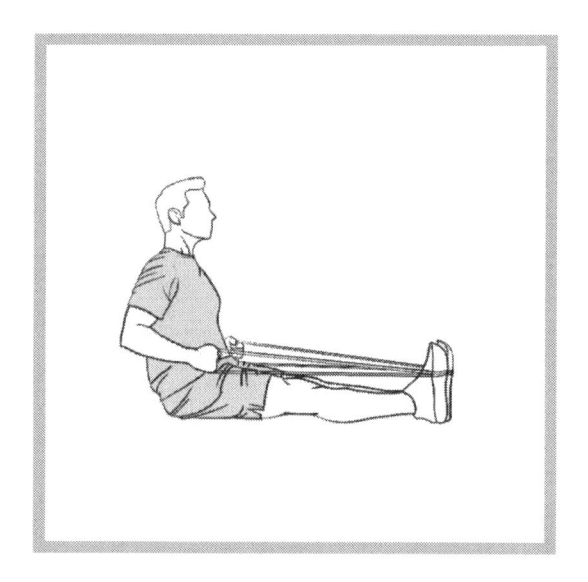

Ankle Pull (Band Stretch)

This stretch will help loosen up the ankle.

Instructions:

- Sit on the floor with your legs straight out in front.
- Take a small towel or resistance and place it around your foot.
- Pull at the band, bringing your foot towards you.
- Hold for 10 seconds, then release, repeat the ten to fifteen times. Repeat on the other foot.

Toe Grip Challenges

This exercise will help to add strength to the muscles on your feet and toes.

Instructions:

- You can use something like a towel or a small object like marbles to help you with this.
- Place the object on the floor and try and grip it with your toes.
- Repeat this gripping motion at least ten times, then repeat on the other foot.

MASSAGE BALLS AND FOAM ROLLERS

I'm sure we have all experienced some sort of tightness in our muscles that makes us stiff and uncomfortable. This is not pleasant, and we want to get rid of this as quickly as possible so we can get our full range of motion back. Luckily there are a few tools that we can use to aid us in this. The massage ball and foam roller have been specifically designed to work out stiffness and knots in our muscles.

The connective tissue in your body that attaches your muscles, bones, and ligament is called fascia, and when they get tight, it is what usually causes this stiffness, you may be feeling. When this happens, knots and trigger points form that cause pain; the best way to get rid of them is to massage

USE IT OR LOSE IT

them out; this is called self-myofascial release. This is where the massage ball and foam rollers come in. If you don't want to go out and buy a massage ball, a tennis ball will work just fine.

Identify the area that has the knot or sore spot. Then, get either your ball or foam roller. You will want to lay down on the object or place it on a wall and gently rock back and forth over the knot; the pressure will help massage it out. Foam rollers work best for larger areas, and balls target very specific areas. Doing this regularly will prevent injuries and future discomfort. It is also an effective way to lengthen and warm up the muscles before stretching.

If you do have the budget to spend a bit more cash on something that will really benefit you through massages and getting out knots, then I would recommend getting a TheraGun. It uses a combination of force and vibrations to relieve pain and stiffness; it can also vastly increase your range of motion. It does all of this without you having to put in anywhere near as much effort as mentioned with massage balls, foam rollers.

3

REPETITIONS: STRETCHING ROUTINES THAT MAKE YOU RECOVER FASTER

Most of us will have at least a few minor muscle injuries or sprains in our lifetime. These can come from exercise, general life, lack of flexibility, or an illness. It is pretty much inevitable, but there are specific routines that can help us overcome these faster, so we don't have to be stuck in that position for a long time.

ROUTINES FOR SPRAINS, INJURIES, ACHES AND PAINS

Minor injuries and sprains, while may not be very serious, can cause some problems and slow us down quite a bit. Let's take a look at a few routines that can help us recover from these specific injuries quicker.

Calf Routine

This is a common injury that occurs when you put too much force on your calf muscle or overstretch it. Take a look at the routine below that will help. You do not have to do all these at once, that might put too much strain on your muscle. Rather start with the first few and then keep adding on more exercises as you get stronger.

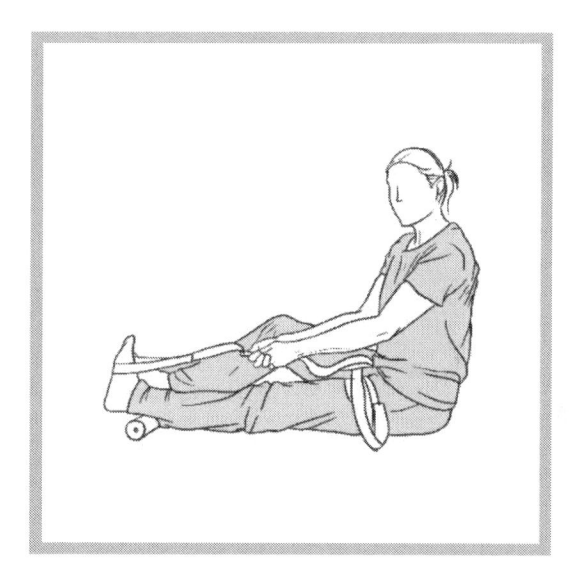

Calf Stretch 1:

- Sit down on the ground with your legs out in front of you.

- Place a roll or rolled-up towel under your ankle to elevate it.
- Grab a strap or belt and place it on your top part of your foot, just below the toes.
- Pull with the strap until you feel the stretch. You might feel a little bit of pain but not too much.
- Hold for 30 seconds and repeat three times.

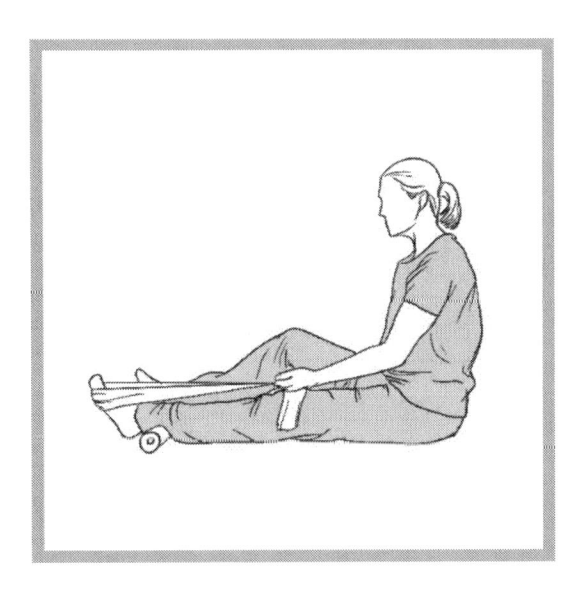

Calf Stretch 2:

- Grab a resistance band, choose the lowest resistance, and place that on the ball of your foot. The roll or towel is still under your ankle.
- Push your toes forward against the resistance band.

- Then slowly bring your foot back up, use controlled movements.
- Repeat ten times at first. If you can, then increase your reps to about fifteen or twenty.

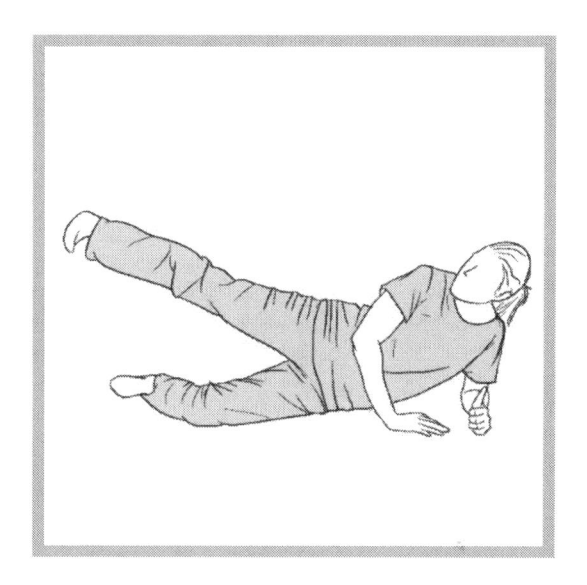

Calf Stretch 3:

- Lay down on your side, bend your bottom leg backward and lift your top leg slightly off the ground.
- Flex your foot, you should feel it in your calf. Point your toe slightly to the floor.
- Pick your leg up and back in one motion; you don't have to lift it too high.

- Bring your leg back down in one controlled movement.
- Start by doing ten to fifteen and then increase if it is easy for you. You may add some weights if you need something extra.

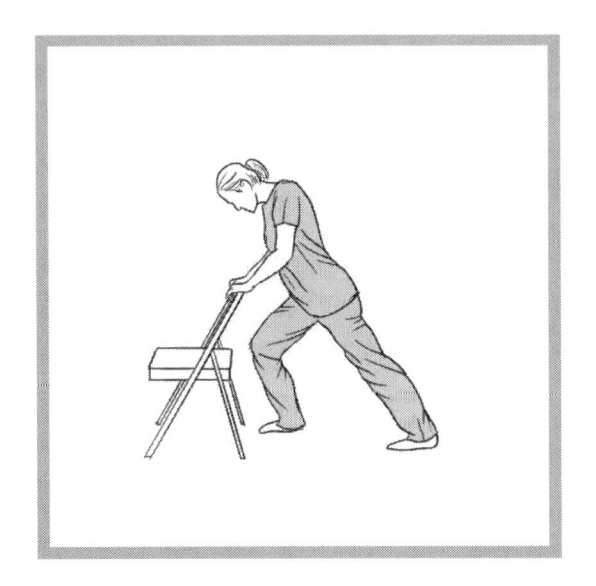

Calf Stretch 4:

- Grab a chair and hold onto the back.
- Take a step back with one leg so that it's stretched out behind you. The other leg should be slightly bent in front of you. Toes pointed forward.
- Lean into your front leg. Hold for 30 seconds and repeat three times.

USE IT OR LOSE IT

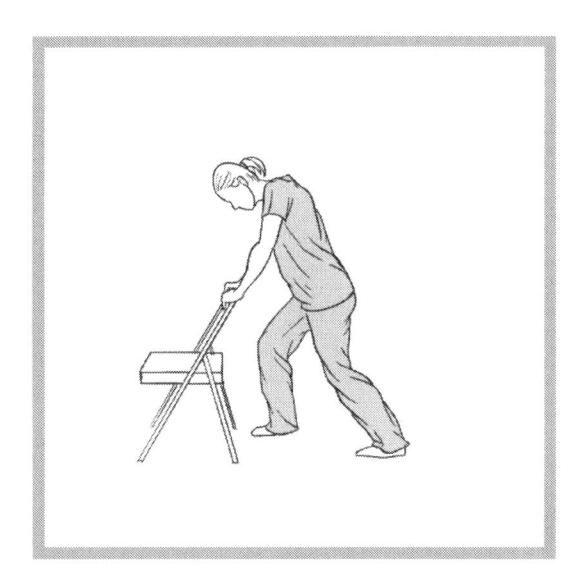

Calf Stretch 5:

- Start in the same position as the previous exercise, but instead of having a straight back leg, just bend it slightly.
- Then lean in and stretch out the muscle. This stretch targets the soleus muscle just below the calf, that's where you should feel it.
- Hold for 30 seconds and repeat three times.

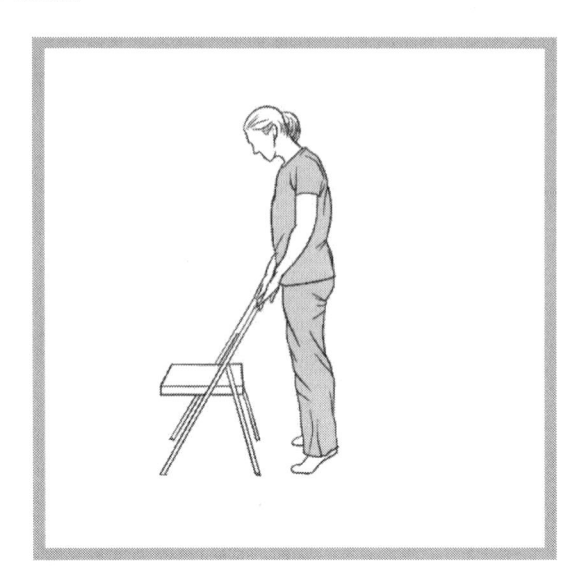

Calf Stretch 6:

- Follow the instructions for the Tip Toe Tense stretch mentioned in the previous chapter.
- Start with about ten repetitions and increase it if you feel you can.

The following exercises are a bit more intense, only do these towards the end of your recovery when you feel that your muscle has strengthened up a bit.

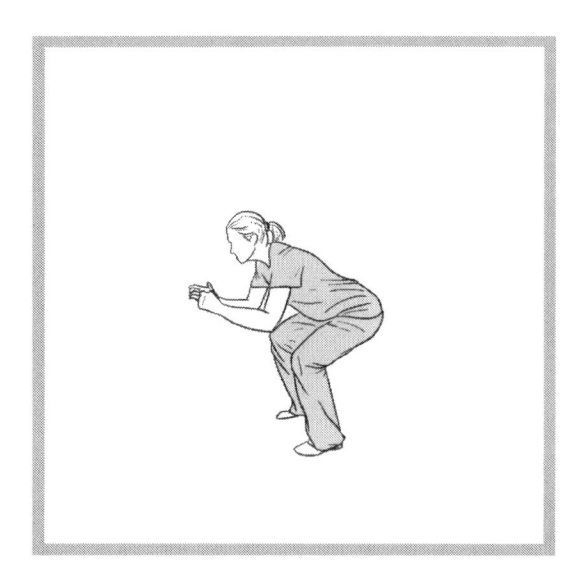

Calf Stretch 7:

- Get into a squat position and lower yourself down into a squat.
- When you bring yourself back up, extend the movement until you are on your toes.
- This should all be one controlled and fluid motion.
- Start with doing five and work your way up.

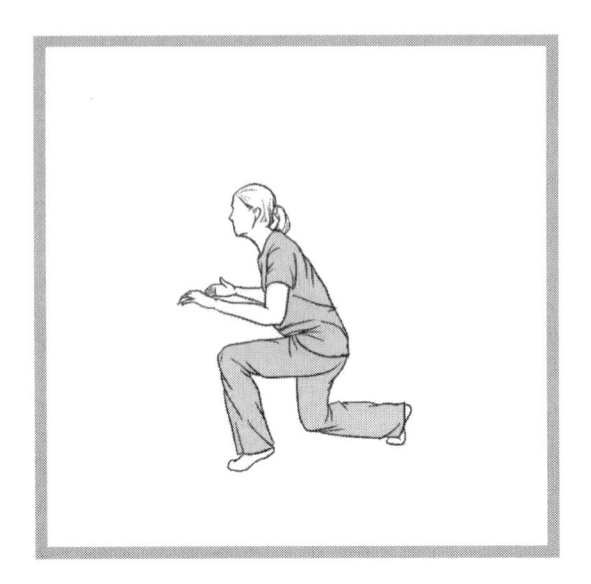

Calf Stretch 8:

- Get into a lunge position—one foot in front and the other behind.
- Get up on your toes on both feet.
- Bend your back knee down, and then bring yourself back up again.
- This should be in one fluid motion.
- Start with five, and when you are comfortable, increase the number you do.

Hamstring Routine

Hamstrings are a common muscle that can get quite tight and get pulled or injured during exercise. If you have a hamstring injury, then the following routine will help you to start recovering.

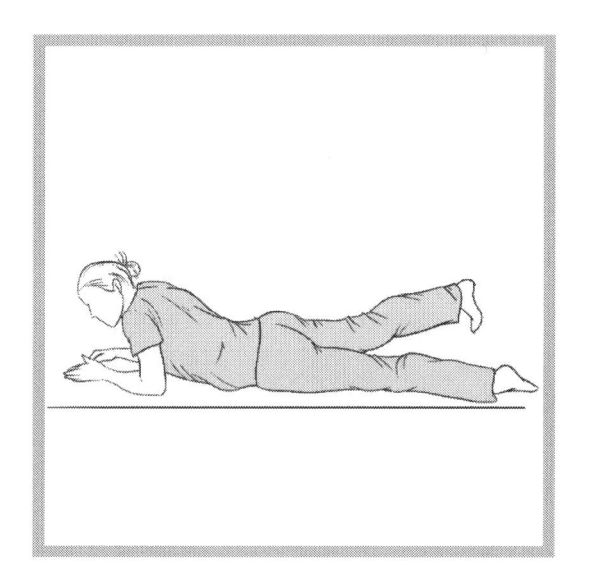

Hamstring Stretch 1:

- Lay down on your belly, prop your body up with your elbows.
- Lift one of your feet as high as you can and then lower it down in one smooth motion.
- Do about ten and see if you can increase it from there.

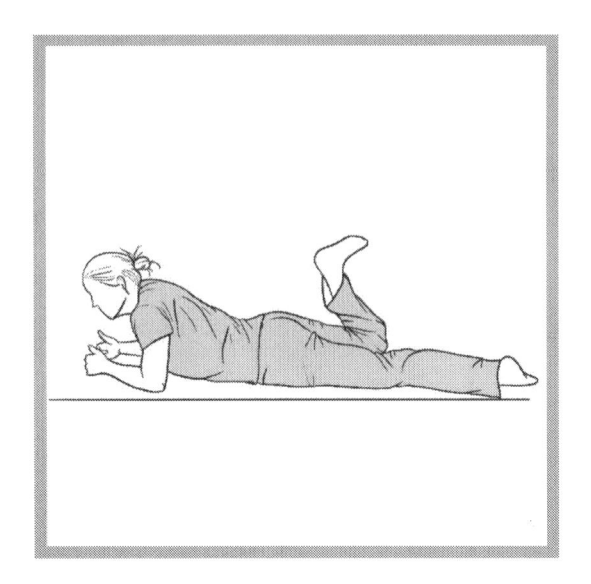

Hamstring Stretch 2:

- Stay on your belly and lift the foot so that it moves towards your butt.
- Keep the motion slow and controlled.
- Start with ten and then add on if you think you can do more.

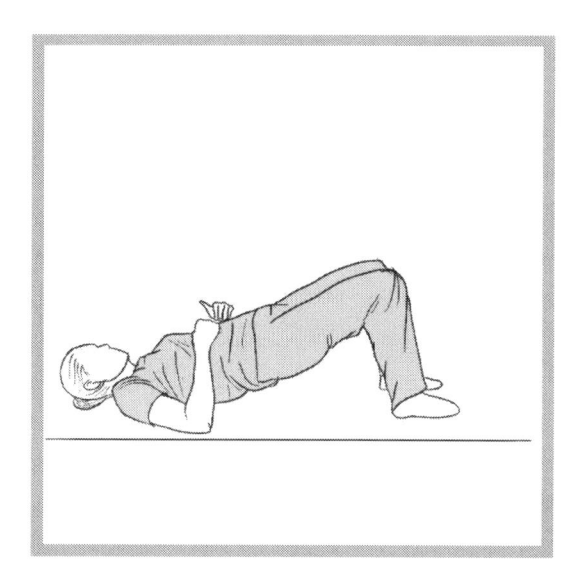

Hamstring Stretch 3:

- Roll over onto your back and bend your knees.
- Lift your hips off the ground and then slowly bring it down.
- Start with ten and then work your way up.
- Make it harder by completing the single-leg version

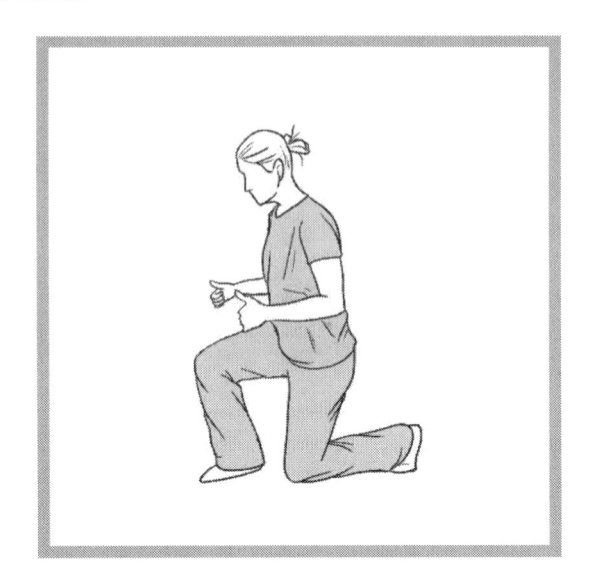

Hamstring Stretch 4:

- Get into a lunge position and just proceed to do a simple lunge.
- Bring your body down and up in one smooth movement, do this slowly.
- Do ten and then work your way up if you can.

Quad Routine

Quads usually get strained when too much force is exerted on it, often due to sports or inflexibility. If you have a pulled quad, do the following routine a few times a day until it heals up.

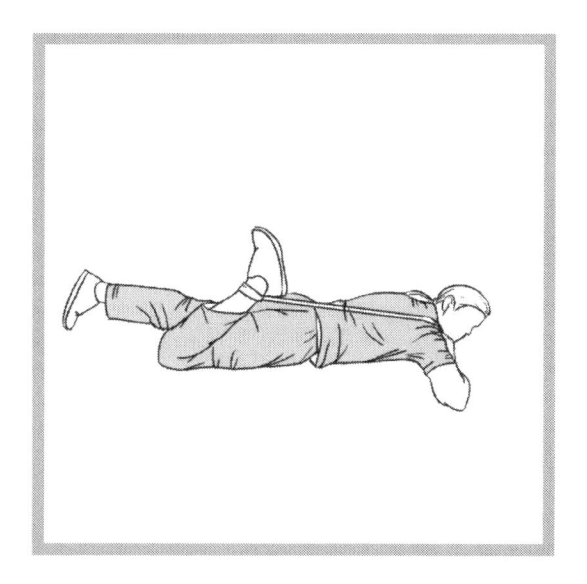

Quad Stretch 1:

- Lay down on your belly and either grab your ankle or use a belt to hold onto your ankle as you pull it towards your butt.
- Pull as far as you can, hold for 30 seconds. Repeat this three times.

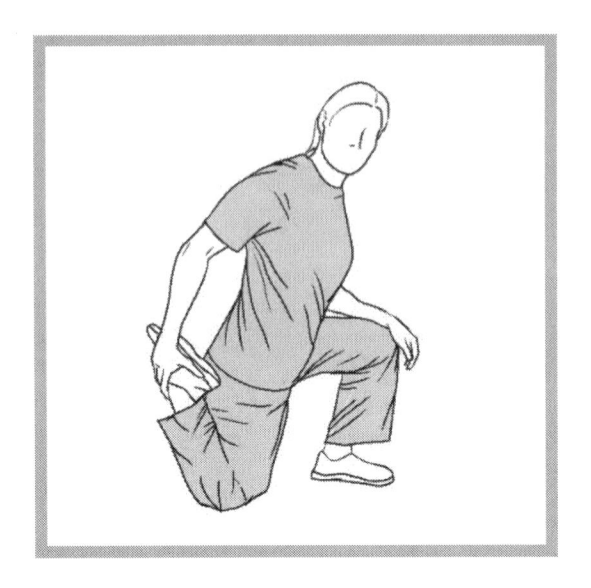

Quad Stretch 2:

- Get on your knees and place one foot in front of you, bent at a 90-degree angle.
- Grab your back foot and bring it up towards your butt, if you would like more of a stretch lean into your front leg.
- Hold for 30 seconds and repeat this three times.

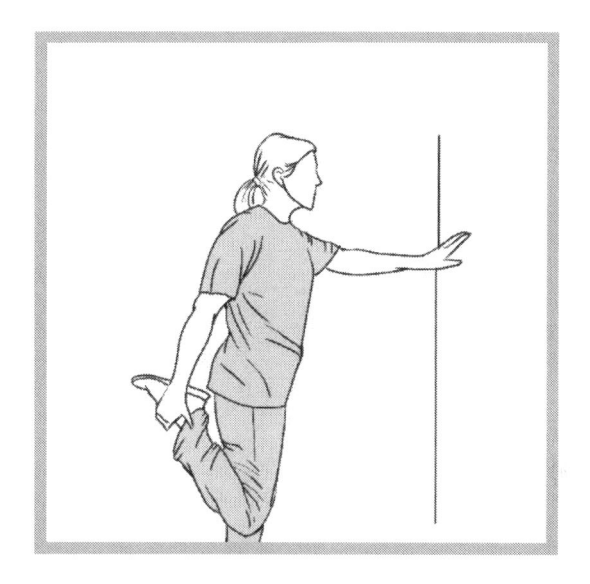

Quad Stretch 3:

- Stand up with your back straight.
- Bend the foot so that it moves toward your butt, grab the foot with your hand and pull it into your butt.
- Make sure both of your knees are still in line.
- Hold for 30 seconds and repeat three times.

Glute Strain

Glute strain can happen from too much sitting or exercising funny. If you have a strain on your glute muscles, follow this routine.

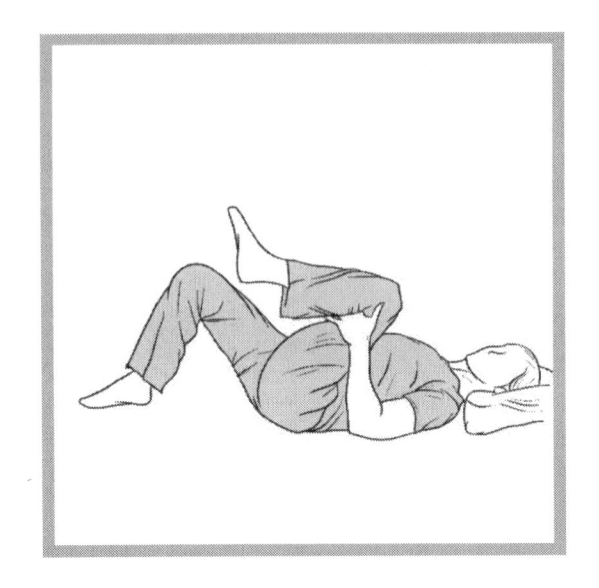

Glute Stretch 1:

- Lay down on your back with your knees bent, grab under your thigh and pull it closer to your body.
- You should feel the stretch in your glute.
- Hold for 30 seconds, repeat three times on each side.

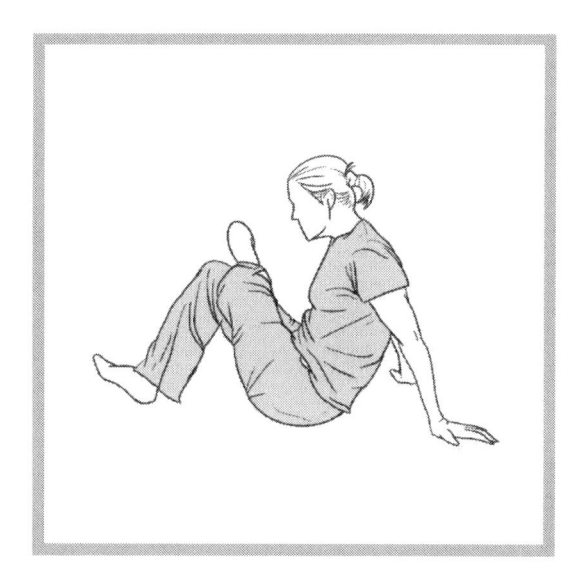

Glute Stretch 2:

- Follow the instructions for the Lying Figure 4 Stretch mentioned in the previous chapter.
- If you want more of a stretch instead of lying down, do it sitting up.
- Use your hands as support behind you and use the leg on the ground to move the bent leg closer to your chest.
- Hold for 30 seconds, repeat three times on each side.

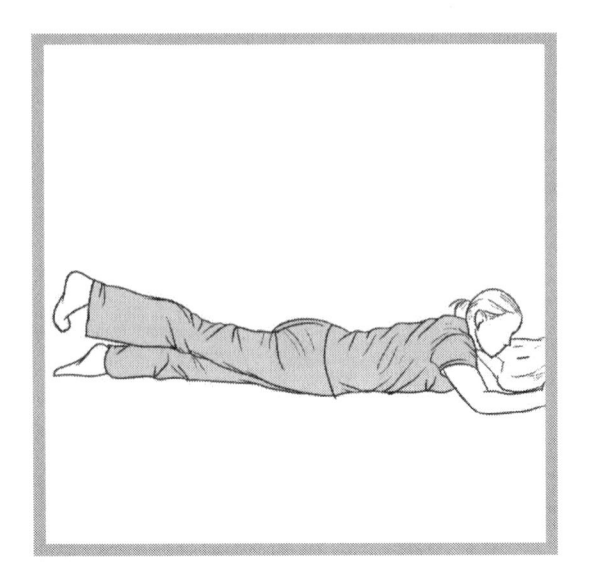

Glute Stretch 3:

- Lay down on your belly, squeeze your butt in tight.
- Lift your leg back.
- Hold for 3 seconds, relax and then repeat ten times.

Groin Strains

A groin strain is a strain on the adductor muscles in your legs. They are positioned in the inner thigh if you have a groin strain use the following routine.

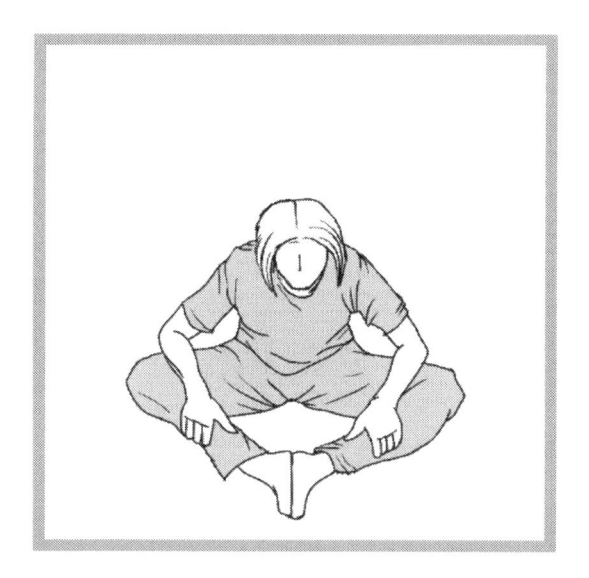

Groin Stretch 1:

- Sit down on the floor and bring your feet together, so the soles of the feet are touching.
- Take your elbows and push down on your inner thighs.
- Lean forward towards your feet.
- Hold for 30 seconds and repeat three times.
- If you want more of a stretch in your inner thigh, pull your feet closer to you.

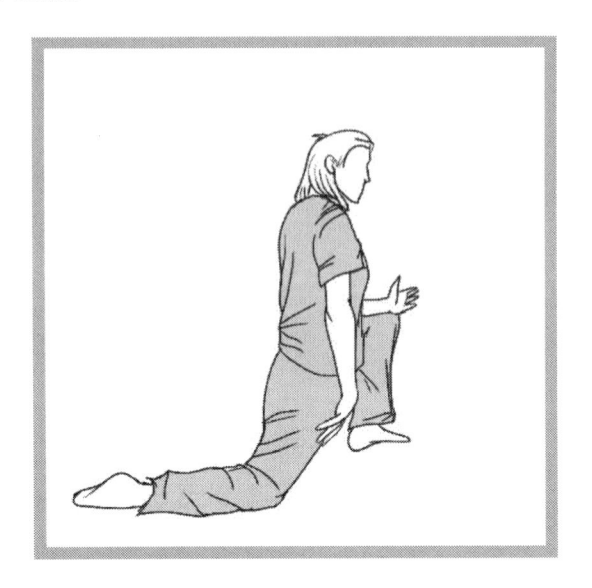

Groin Stretch 2:

- Get down on one knee with the other leg in front of you.
- Move that leg to the side, as far as it is comfortable for you.
- Push forward with your hips.
- Hold for 30 seconds and repeat three times on each leg.

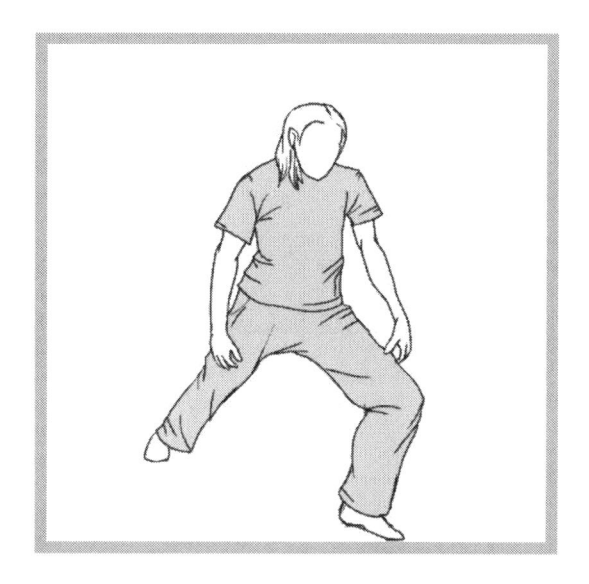

Groin Stretch 3:

- Stand up straight and step your foot forward and to the outside in a 45-degree angle.
- Push yourself forward into your front leg.
- Hold for 30 seconds and repeat three times.

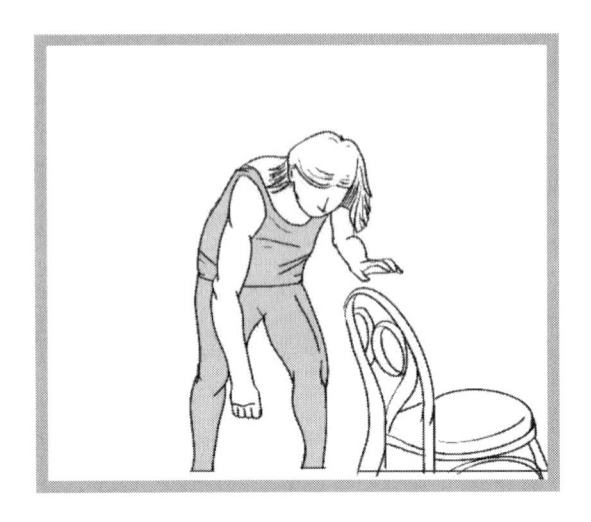

Shoulder Pain

If we put too much weight on our shoulders or funnily sleep on our shoulders, it can cause shoulder pain. If you suffer from shoulder pain, follow this routine.

Shoulder Stretch 1:

- Bend down and hold onto a chair, let your arm hang down in front of you.
- Swing your body around like a pendulum; your whole body should be moving, not just your arm.
- If you want your shoulder to open up a bit more, hold a weight in your hand.
- Do this for a few minutes.

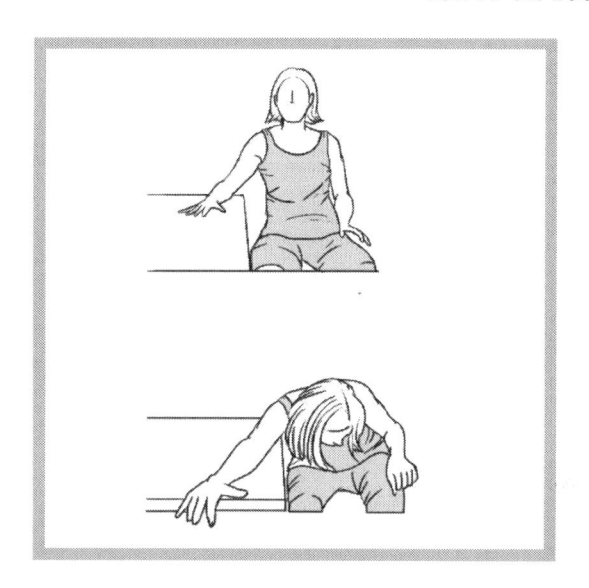

Shoulder Stretch 2:

- Sit at a table and place your forearm on the surface.
- Slide the arm forward and backward on the table to open up the shoulder.
- Then do the same movement at a 45-degree angle on the table.
- Move on to sliding in circles if those feel good.
- Repeat as many times as desired.

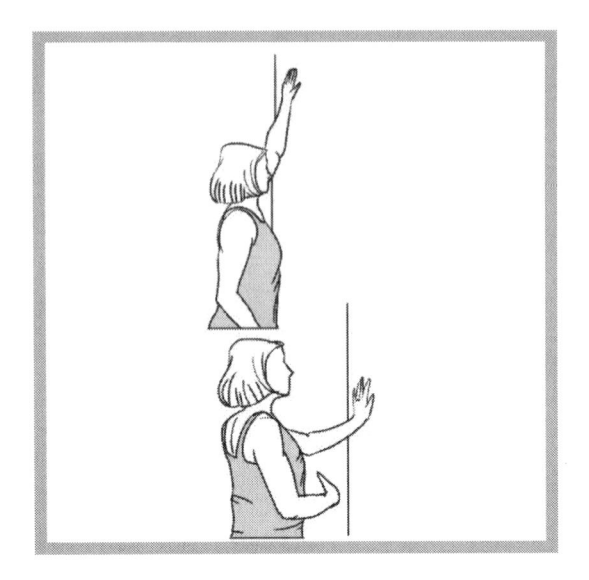

Shoulder Stretch 3:

- Place your hand on a wall.
- Slide it up and once you get pretty high lean into the wall.
- Bring your hand back down.
- Repeat as many times as desired.

Rotator Cuff Stain

The rotator cuff surrounds the shoulder and is made up of muscles and tendons. If you have injured your rotator cuff, then follow this routine. You may also incorporate the shoulder routine above and vice versa.

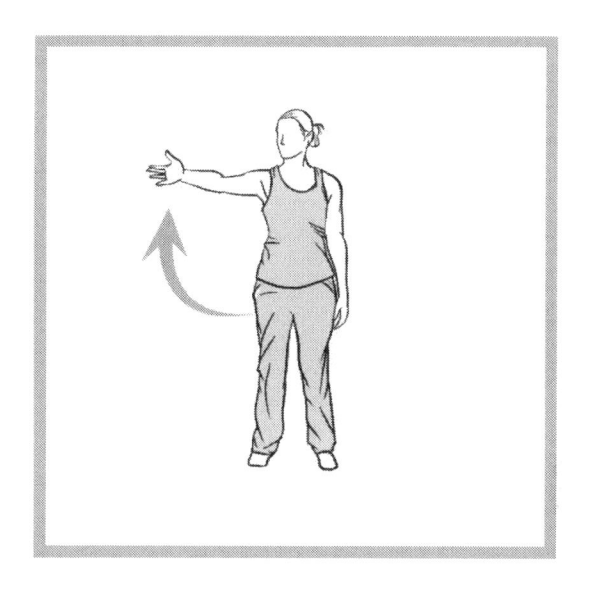

Rotator Cuff Stretch 1:

- Stand up straight with your arm just slightly in front of you facing 45 degrees to the side.
- With a straight arm, lift it to about 90 degrees and bring it down again.
- Use controlled movements.
- Repeat as many times as desired.

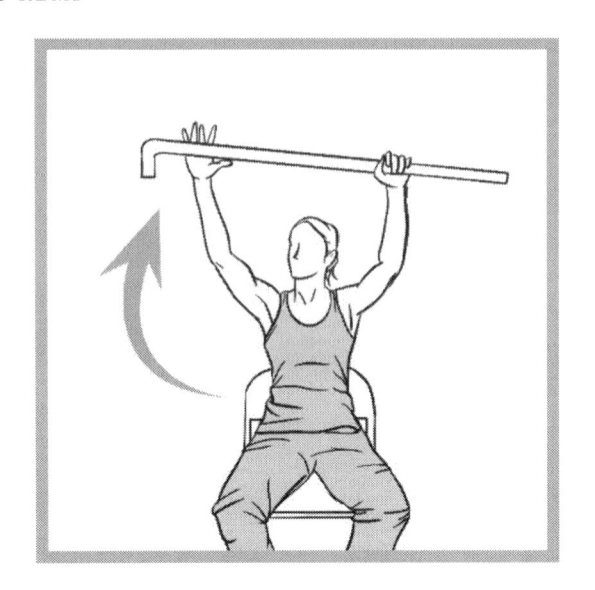

Rotator Cuff Stretch 2:

- Sit down on a chair and have either a stick or a pipe in hand.
- The injured side is just going to rest on the stick, and the other hand will be doing all the work.
- Place the hand of the injured side on the stick, lift the stick with the other hand until it is just over your head.
- Slowly bring it back down.
- Repeat as many times as desired.

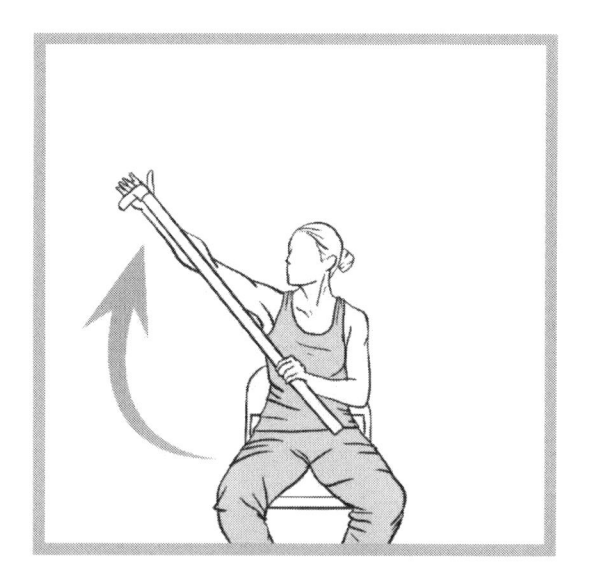

Rotator Cuff Stretch 3:

- This is the same principle as stretch 2. The injured hand is just resting while the other one is doing the work.
- Place the hand of the injured arm on the side of the stick or pipe and use your other hand to push it to the side.
- Repeat as many times as desired.

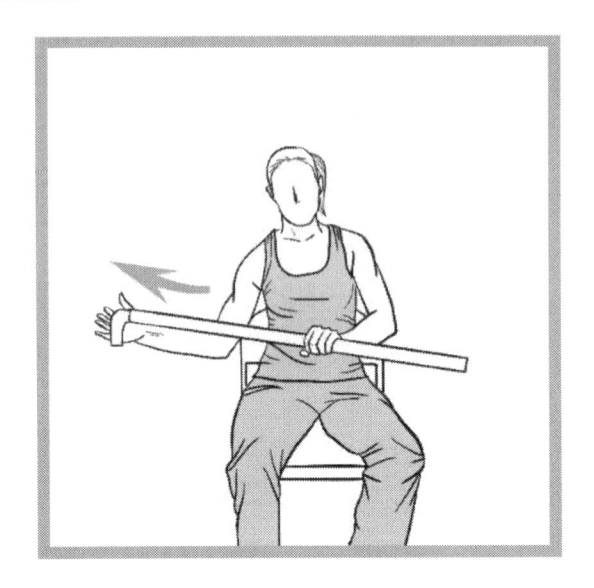

Rotator Cuff Stretch 4:

- Still using the pipe or stick, hold the hand of your injured side at a 90-degree angle with your fingers facing forward.
- Use the pipe or stick to push the hand back. The motion is the same as that of a door opening and closing.
- Repeat as many times as desired.

You may also want to refer to the shoulder pain exercises.

Knee and Hip Strain

Knee and hip injuries can occur for many different reasons,

but they can be quite debilitating if not attended to. Use the following routine to ease any discomfort in these areas.

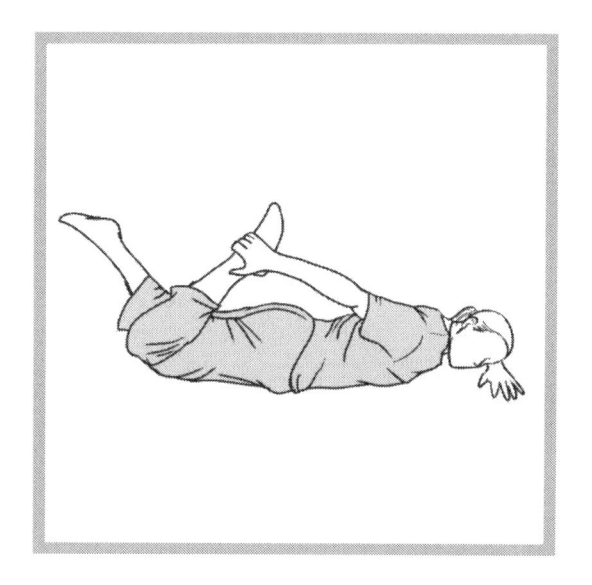

Knee and Hip Stretch 1:

- Lay down on the ground with your belly facing the floor.
- Put your face down on the ground and take your arm around your back to grab your foot.
- Pull your leg up off the ground; your shoulder can be off the ground as well.
- Hold for 30 seconds and repeat three times.

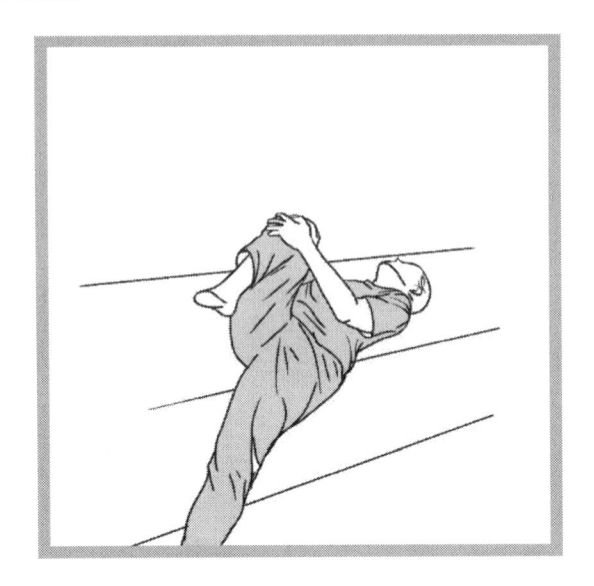

Knee and Hip Stretch 2:

- Lay down on the edge of a bed. Your injured side should be hanging off the side of the bed. Be careful that you don't slip off.
- Grab the shin of your other leg and pull it into your body.
- This stretch allows the hip to stretch using its natural weight.
- Hold for 30 seconds and repeat three times.

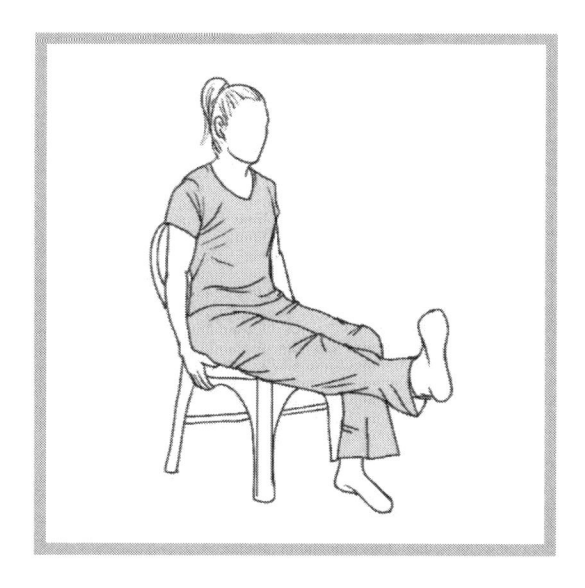

Knee and Hip Stretch 3:

- Sit on a chair with your back straight. You shouldn't be leaning back during this stretch.
- Slowly kick your leg straight out and slowly bring it back down to the ground.
- If it is too easy for you, add some weight to your ankle
- Repeat ten to fifteen times and increase as you get stronger.

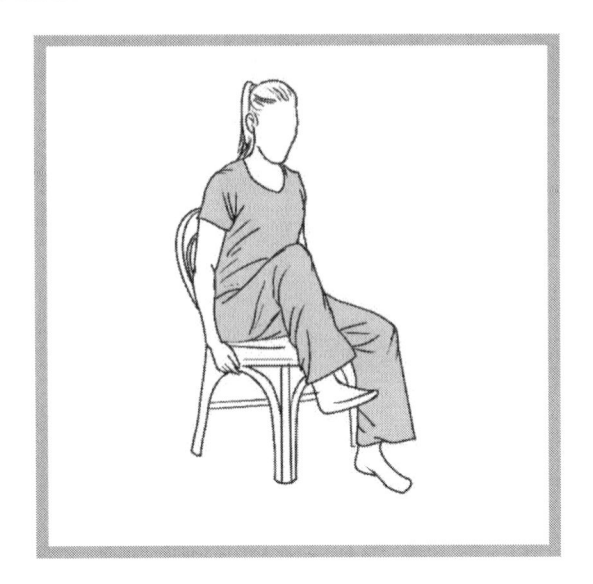

Knee and Hip Stretch 4:

- Still sitting on your chair, drive your knee up.
- Slowly bring it down. Make sure your movements are controlled.
- This is a hip flexion strengthening move.
- Do this ten to fifteen times and increase as you get stronger.

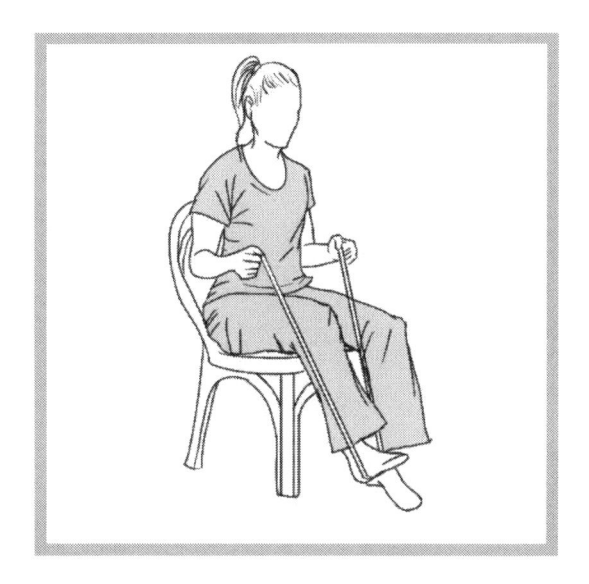

Knee and Hip Stretch 5:

- Grab a resistance band, use the band that is the lowest resistance.
- Place the band in the middle of your foot.
- With controlled movements, lift your knee up and then push down into the resistance band.
- Repeat ten to fifteen times and increase as you get stronger.

Achilles Pain

The Achilles tendon is the tissue that connects the calf muscle to the heel bone. When we have pain in this area, especially if it's constant, it is called Achilles tendinitis.

Follow this routine to help stretch out this area and get it feeling better.

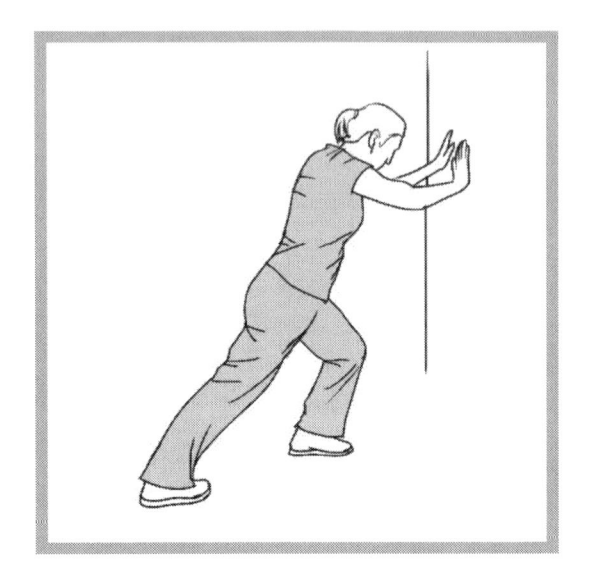

Achilles Stretch 1:

- Start by standing next to a wall; you will be leaning against it.
- Step forward with one leg and have the other one behind you. The leg behind you will be the one being stretched out.
- Make sure your feet are faced towards the wall and are flat on the ground.
- Bend your front left and lean into that leg, so it

moves towards the wall. Keep your back leg straight.
- Hold for 30 seconds and repeat three times.

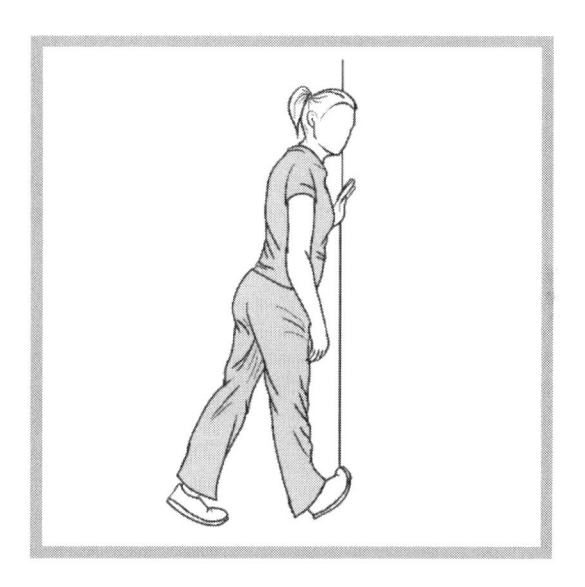

Achilles Stretch 2:

- Get up close to the wall and place your toes on the wall.
- Get your toes as high as you can on the wall while your heel is still on the ground.
- Lean into the wall with your body.
- Hold this for 30 seconds and repeat three times.

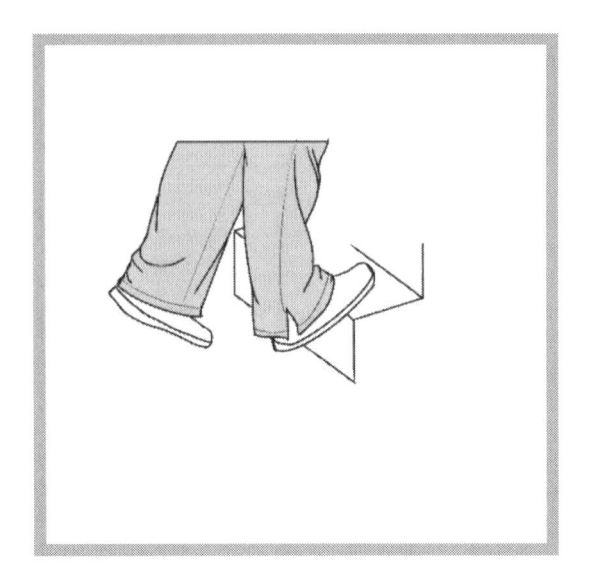

Achilles Stretch 3:

- You will need a step or step ladder for this stretch.
- Place the ball of your foot onto the step and let your heel hang off. Your other foot should also be hanging off the step.
- Drop the heel of your foot as low as you can get it; you will feel the stretch in your Achilles tendon.
- Hold this for 30 seconds and repeat three times.

Back Strains

Many things can cause back strains from lifting heavy weights to having improper posture or even just sleeping in an uncomfortable position. If you have a back strain, then follow this routine to ease that pain.

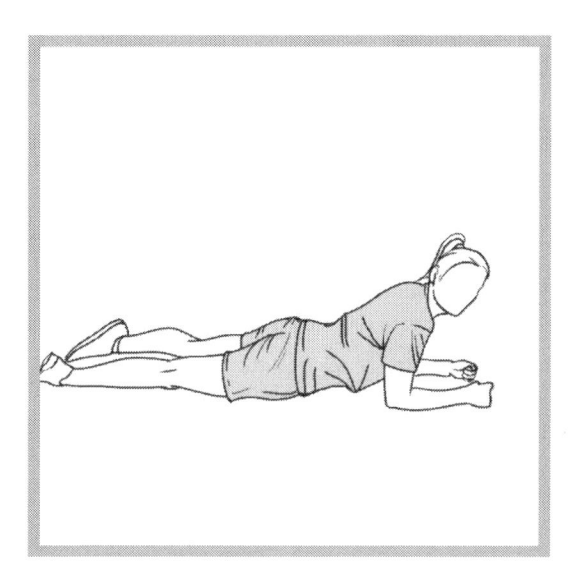

Back Stretch 1:

- Lay down on your belly and prop yourself up on your elbows.
- Your hips should be on the ground, try not to lift your stomach either.
- Hold this position for 30 seconds and repeat three times.

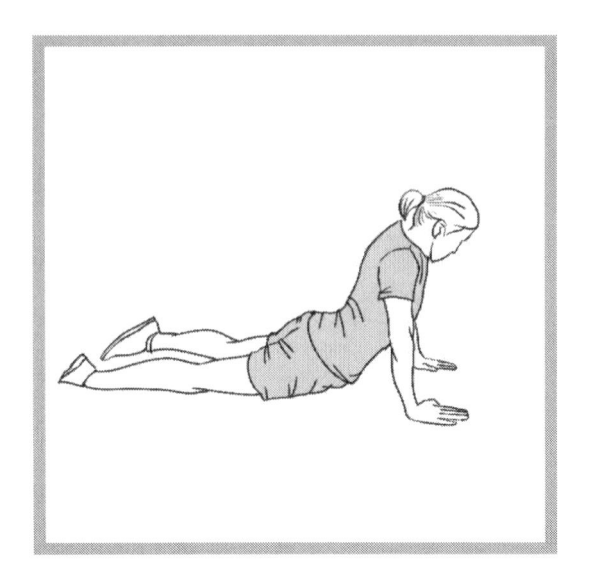

Back Stretch 2:

- This is just a step further from the previous one.
- Lift yourself on your hands, try and keep your hips to the ground.
- Hold this for 30 seconds and repeat three times.

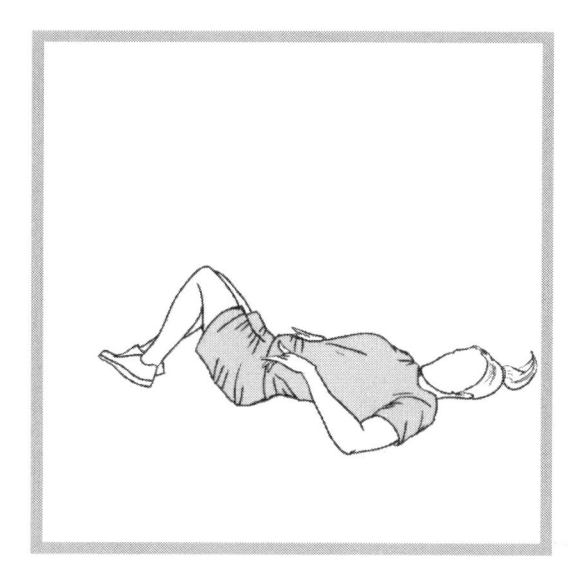

Back Stretch 3:

- Move over onto your back, have your knees pointing to the ceiling.
- Drop your knees to the one side and roll your hips over, before your knees touch the ground start rolling over to the other side.
- Do this ten times or hold for 30 seconds and repeat three times.

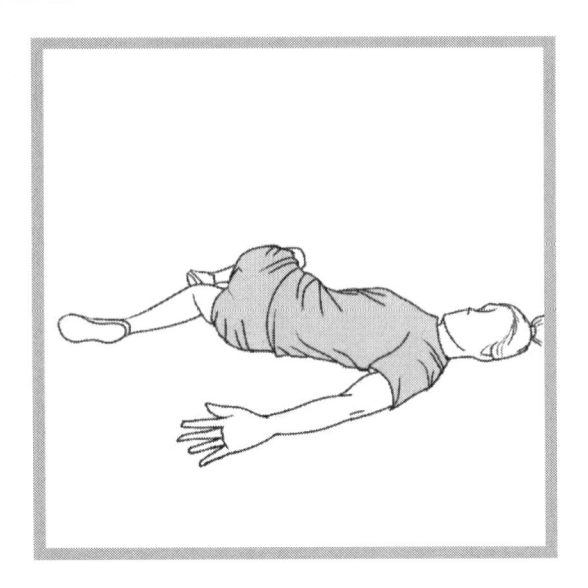

Back Stretch 4:

- This is the next progression from Back Stretch 3.
- When you roll over to one side, drop your knee to the ground and pull it up to a 90-degree angle and drop it to the ground.
- If you want a deeper stretch in your lumbar, take your hand and press down on your top leg.
- Hold for 30 seconds and repeat on the other side.

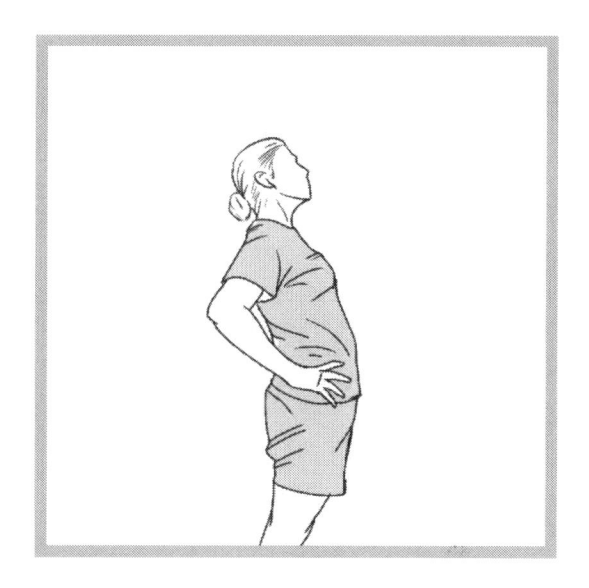

Back Stretch 5:

- Stand up straight and place your hands on your hips.
- Rotate your hips back so that you are looking at the ceiling, the hands-on your hips should give you some support. Don't bend your knees.
- Hold for 30 seconds and repeat three times.

MOBILITY LIMITING ILLNESSES

Joint and muscle pain are most commonly caused by the things we do in our daily lives, but in some cases, pain is caused by illnesses. These illnesses show up usually by no fault of our own; they are just age or genetics. While there may not be anything that we can do to stop ourselves from getting these illnesses, there is something we can do to reduce discomfort significantly. These stretching routines will help ease the discomfort and strengthen the joints and muscles so that you can live a more comfortable life.

Arthritis

Arthritis is pretty common, mostly in older people, but it has been seen in people who are teens and young adults as well. It is most common in the hands, and it can cause joint pain and stiffness. Sometimes it causes redness and swelling in the joint areas. You might also notice your range of mobility has lessened. If you have arthritis, then follow this routine to help relieve the pressure on your joints and strengthen up your hands in the process.

USE IT OR LOSE IT

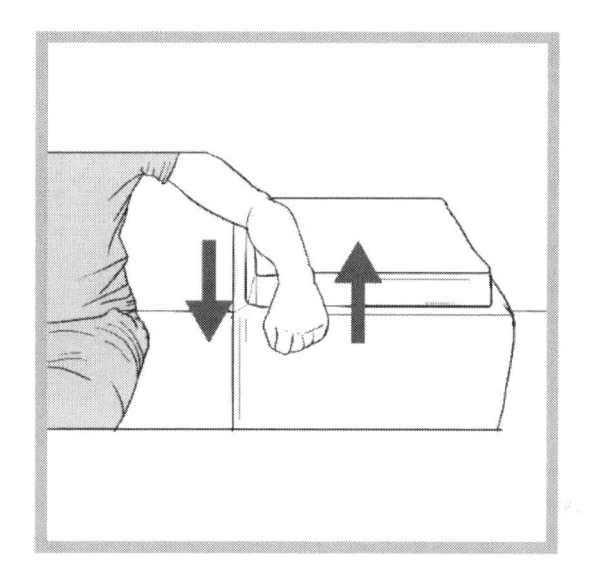

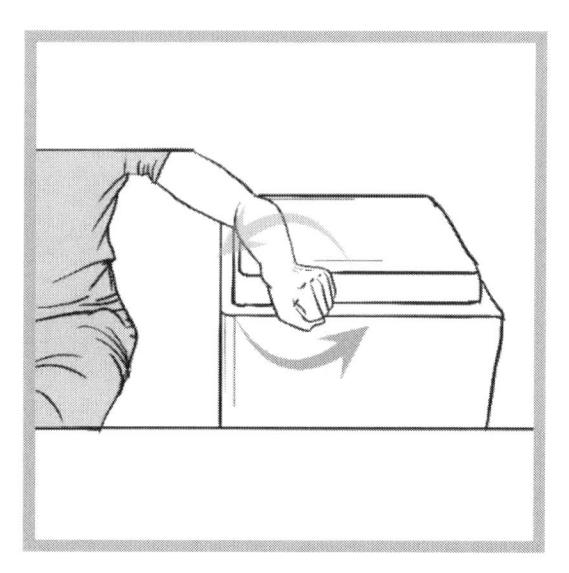

Arthritis Stretch 1:

359

- Prop your arm up on a table or counter. Let your wrist hang off the edge.
- Warm your wrist up by moving it up and down on the edge of the counter. Do this about ten to fifteen times.
- Switch to moving your wrist side to side, also ten to fifteen times.

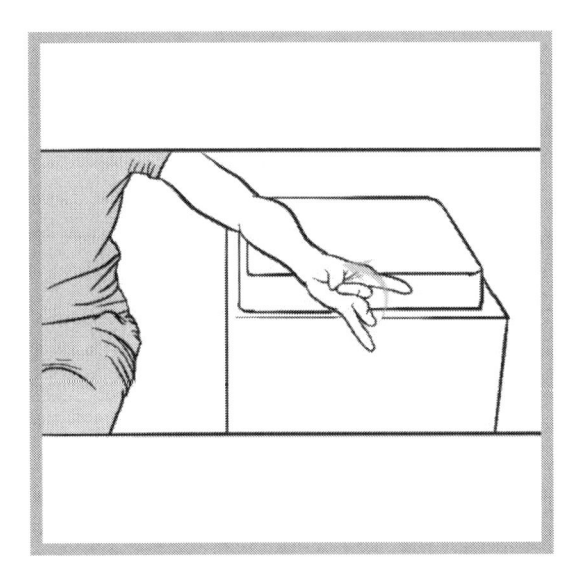

Arthritis Stretch 2:

- Open up your hands like you are showing the number 5.
- Keep your fingers as straight as possible and bring your fingers in one by one to meet your thumb.

This allows the focus to be on the bottom joints of the fingers.

- Repeat this about three times on all your fingers.

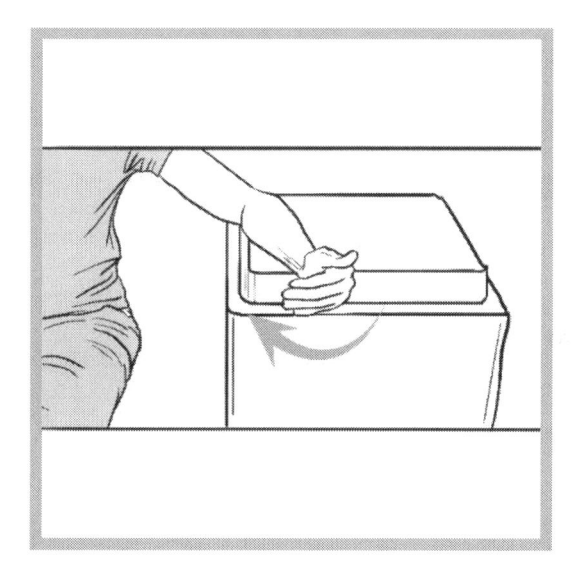

Arthritis Stretch 3:

- Still, with your hand open, stick all your fingers together with the thumb facing up.
- Keeping your fingers straight, bend at the knuckle to try and create a 90-degree angle with your hand. Release and go back to a straight hand.
- Next, focus on the joint just above your knuckle. Bend that in, almost creating a claw. Release and go back to the starting position.

- Next, move to the top joint of the finger. You also want just to move this joint down, this can be difficult, so hold your finger just below the joint and move it down. Do this with each finger.
- Repeat each one of these ten to fifteen times.

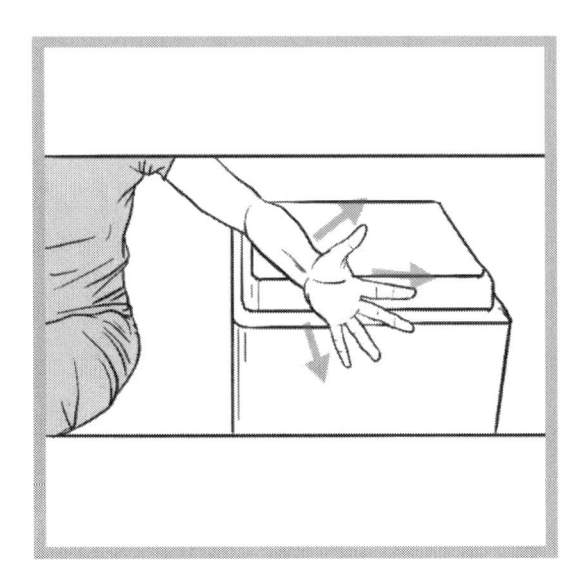

Arthritis Stretch 4:

- Start with your hand open and all your fingers together.
- Fan them out wide, then bring them back together.
- Do this for about 2 minutes a few times a day.
- You may repeat all the stretches in this routine a few times a day to ease any discomfort.

Tendonitis

The inflammation of the tendon causes tendonitis; it is more common in certain people than others. This is just due to genetics or the strain that is being placed on the tendon. If you put too much pressure or use the tendon too much, it can result in tendonitis. If you have tendonitis in your heel, you may follow the routine for stretching out the Achilles tendon that was mentioned above. If you have tendonitis in your wrist, then follow the following routine.

Tendonitis Stretch 1:

- The first stretch in this routine is the same one for Arthritis Stretch 1.
- Do these movements but do them slower and more controlled; you want to feel the stretch in the wrist.
- Do this ten to fifteen times.
- As you get stronger, you can do this with weight. Try a soup can or similar and do the same movements but while holding the can.

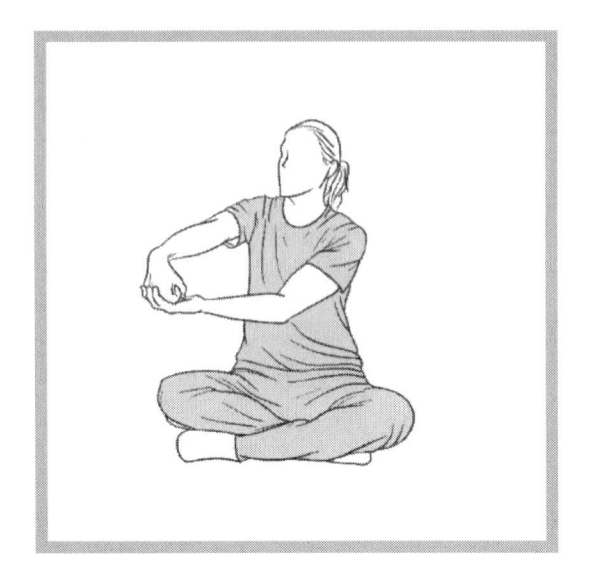

Tendonitis Stretch 2:

- Stretch out your arm in front of you and ball up your fist.
- Bend your wrist downwards and take your other hand and pull it towards you.
- Hold for 30 seconds.
- Open up your hands and flip your wrist upwards.
- Take the other hand, and pull the wrist towards you.
- Hold for 30 seconds.
- Repeat three times each way.
- Another variation would be to put your hands on the ground or wall and lean into it each way. You

should feel all these stretches in your wrists and the tendons running up your forearms.

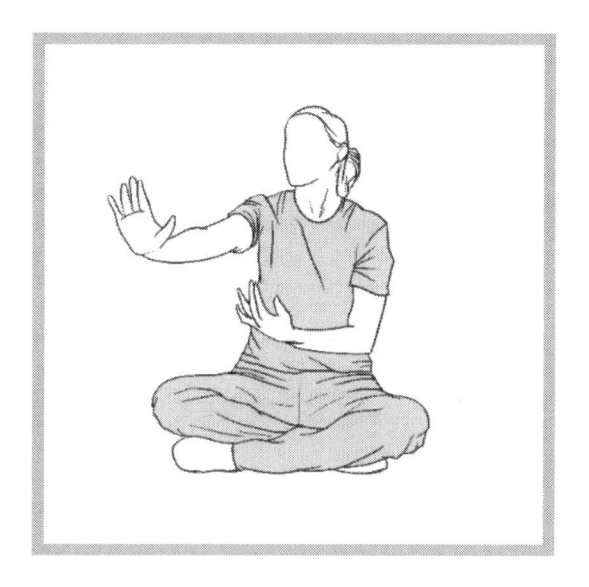

Tendonitis Stretch 3:

- Open up your hands so that your fingers are splayed out.
- Then ball it up into a fist. Repeat as many times as desired.
- You do not need to hold this; the goal is just to get your hand moving.

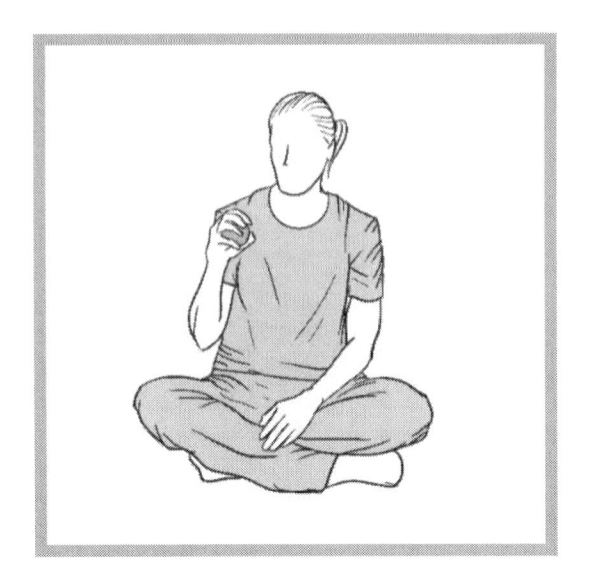

Tendonitis Stretch 4:

- Grab either a stress ball or a tennis ball.
- Squeeze that in your hands for about five to ten seconds.
- Release and repeat five times.
- If you don't have a ball or want something softer, you can use a pool noodle or rolled-up towel.

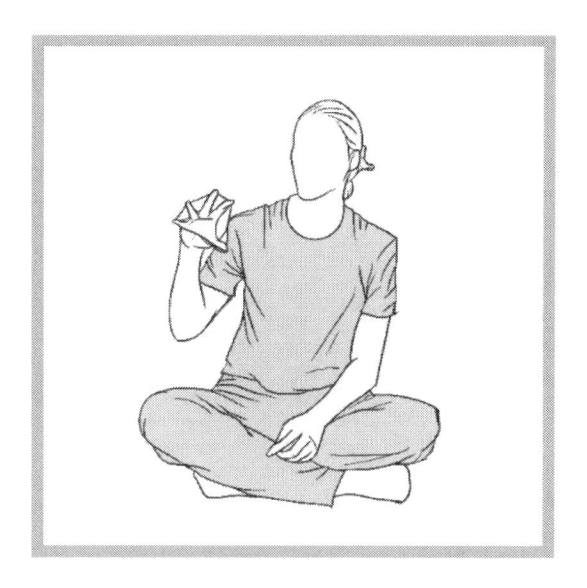

Tendonitis Stretch 5:

- Grab a small rubber band.
- Place it around your fingers and stretch your fingers open and closed.
- Go slow, so the band doesn't pop off.
- You want to repeat this about three times.

Carpal Tunnel Syndrome

Carpal tunnel syndrome is found in the arm and wrist and is a result of a pinched nerve. The symptoms are usually tingling, sensitivity, pain, and numbness. If you suffer from carpal tunnel syndrome, then follow this routine to ease discomfort and pain.

You should feel stretching and tension when doing these stretches, but not any severe pain. You might feel tingling in your fingertips; when you let it up, it should stop. If the tingling does not stop, this is an indication you have gone too far with the stretch. There is too much pressure on the nerve. Also, it might be an indication that there is something else wrong; this would be a good time to check in with your doctor or physician so they can diagnose you accurately.

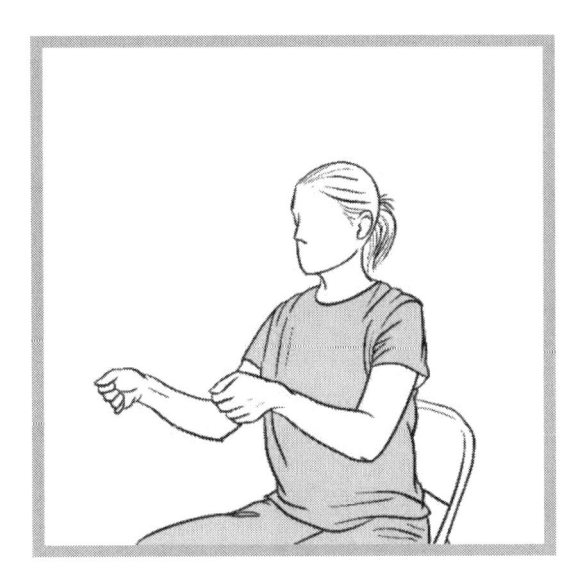

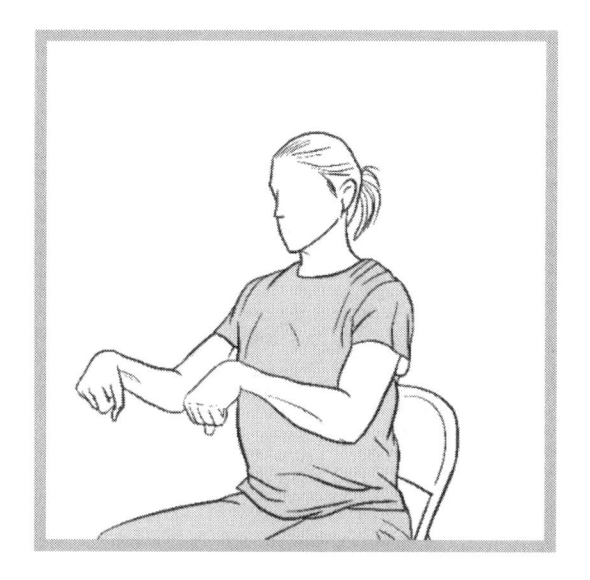

Carpal Tunnel Stretch 1:

- Hold your hands up in front of you, with your fists closed.
- Turn your wrists up, so your knuckles face the ceiling then bring them down to face the floor.
- Repeat ten times up and ten times down.
- Turn your hands to the side, so your thumb is upwards.
- Move your wrist up and then down, if the same motion as before.
- Repeat ten times up and ten times down.
- Make sure you are doing this is a continuous motion.

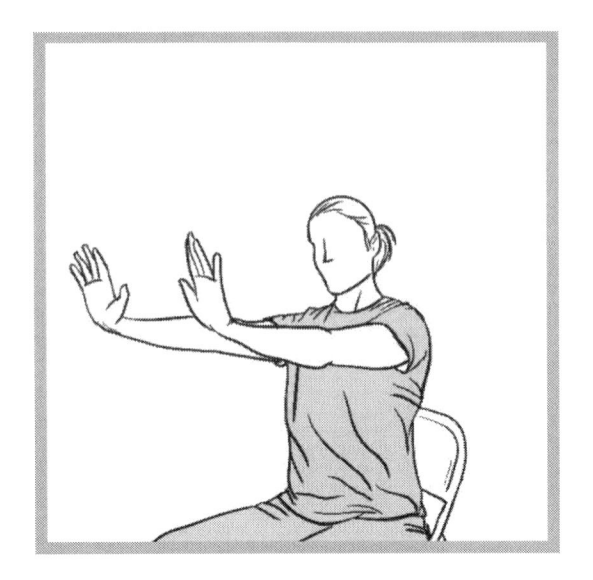

Carpal Tunnel Stretch 2:

- Stretch your arms out straight in front of you. Your hands should be open.
- Turn your wrists up so that your fingers point upwards.
- If you need less of a stretch, close your fingers. If you want more of a stretch, push your hands up against a wall.
- Hold for 30 seconds and repeat three times.

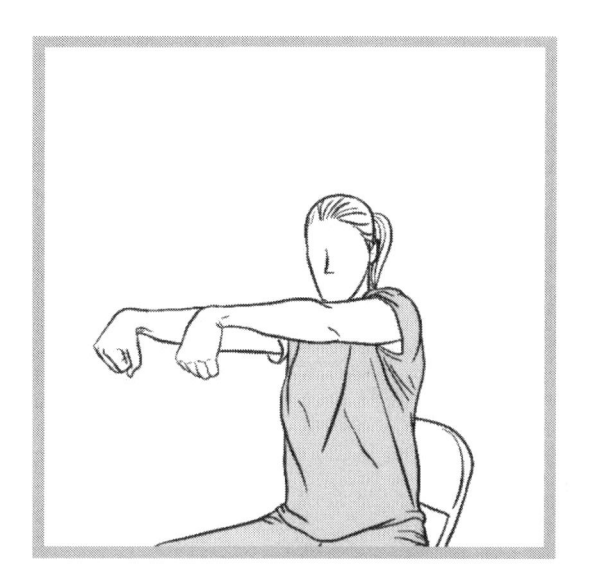

Carpal Tunnel Stretch 3:

- Still have your arms stretched out in front of you. Flip your wrists downward and curl your fingers in.
- If you want less of a stretch, then open up your fingers. If you want more of a stretch, then press your hands up against a wall.
- Hold for 30 seconds and repeat three times.

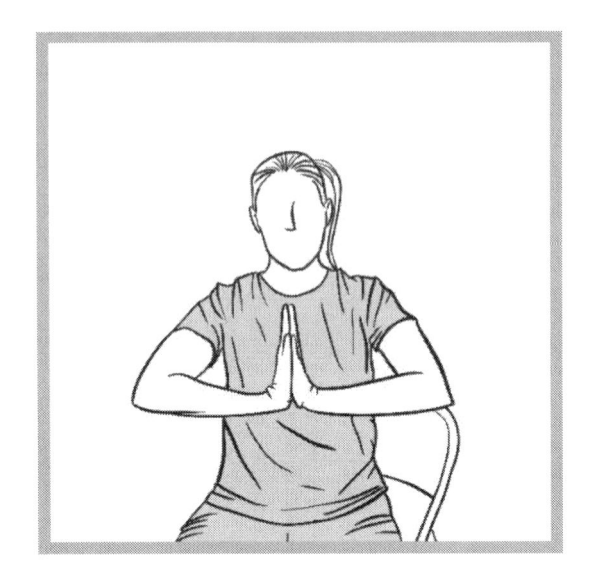

Carpal Tunnel Stretch 4:

- Place your palms together in a praying formation.
- Bring your wrists down, and at the same time, your elbows should be moving outwards.
- Push down as low as you can.
- Hold for 30 seconds and repeat three times.

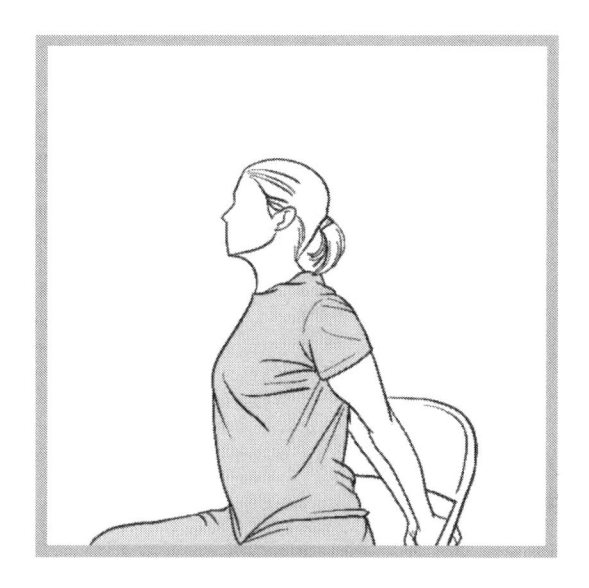

Carpal Tunnel Stretch 5:

- Clasp your hands behind you.
- Push your hands down and push your chest out.
- Hold for 30 seconds and repeat three times.
- This is more of a peck stretch, but it is good because that whole area is connected, so it would still be beneficial to you.

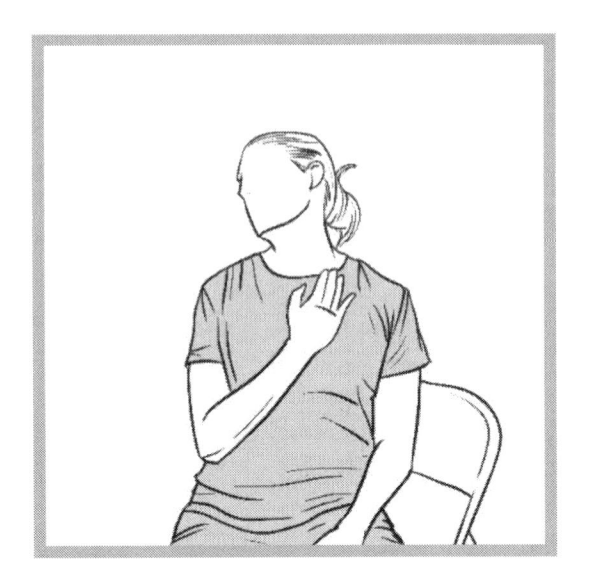

Carpal Tunnel Stretch 6:

- Hold your hand up to the side of your chest on a 90-degree angle. Your hand should be almost parallel to your head.
- Keep pressure on your upper chest and tilt your head the opposite side to your hand.
- Repeat ten times. Do this on the other side.
- This stretch is done to glide the nerve out, and it is not necessary to do it multiple times a day, since it could irritate the area.

4

THE FINAL PUSH: STRETCHING ROUTINES TO OPTIMIZE YOUR WORKOUTS

We have already chatted about the many benefits stretching has for your body and general life. But it can really improve the quality of your workouts as well. When you work out, your muscles are constantly flexing and contracting; they are in a constant state of movement. If you have limited flexibility, you will have limited muscle movement, which will put a cap on your workouts and progress.

Stretching also increases your rate of recovery after a workout. When we stretch, we increase blood circulation; this results in more nutrients being available for the muscles and a faster removal of harmful waste. You will ultimately feel better because of this. Stretching also provides you with a wider range of motion, which means the moves you perform can be more dynamic. No matter how far along you are in your fitness journey, stretching is a good weapon to have in your arsenal to increase your athletic development.

Using stretching in tandem with a workout is an extremely effective way to stay young and healthy. They tend to feed into each other; stretching improves your workouts or exercise, and that improves your health, and the cycle can then repeat.

GET THE MOST OUT OF YOUR STRETCH

As an athlete or avid gym-goer, you want to be able to get the most out of everything you do, and as with everything there is a right way and a wrong way to stretch. To reap all the benefits from stretching, you need to be mindful of a few things. The first thing is that stretching causes tension but not pain. That hurts so good feeling is normal; this shows that you are engaging those muscles, but any uncomfortable or piercing pain is an indication that you should stop. Pain can either be an indication that you have done the stretch wrong or that your muscles are not ready for that move as yet. Flexibility is built up over time, so don't rush it.

The second thing to remember is to breathe. Sometimes when we are so focused on the exercise or stretch, we forget that we need to breathe, when we hold our breath, our muscles tense up. We want our muscles to be as loose as possible when stretching, so remember to inhale and exhale constantly.

The third thing you need to keep in mind when it comes to stretching is that it is not a warm-up. In fact, your muscles should be warmed up for you to get the best out of your stretches. Cold muscles limit your movement and might even lead to injuries. The best way to warm up your muscles is a light 5 to 10-minute jog, either outside or on a treadmill. This will start activating your muscles and get them ready for your routine.

The final thing to remember when stretching is that you should not be bouncing. Stretching is about fluid motions, not stop-start or pulsing movements. Stretching is usually measured by the seconds you hold it for rather than how many you do, so if you are moving too quickly so that you can get to the next one, you will not get the most out of your stretch. Try and move as smoothly as possible; remember to relax and enjoy the moments.

ROUTINES FOR TARGETED AREAS

Every part of your body is different, and when it comes to stretching, each one has different requirements and a varied range of motion. I have broken up the stretching routines into sections; you will be able to partner stretching routines with the parts of your body you are working out that day. This way, you will be able to get the best results from your stretching and your workouts.

After each routine, you are encouraged to take a few minutes to connect with your body, engaging in a time of mindfulness. You can do this by lying down on your back and taking deep breaths. Think about how you feel and how the stretches made the different parts of your body feel. You may even find it helpful to touch the areas you are thinking about physically. The goal here is to increase the mind-body connection. If you know your body, you will be able to pick up on things faster.

Upper Body Routine

Having tight shoulders or a tight chest will diminish your range of motion, and you will lose some of the quality of your workout. Flexibility will help you get better results in any section of your upper body. They are all connected, and that is why it is essential not to neglect stretching out your entire upper body. Follow this routine to help you benefit from the flexibility of your upper body.

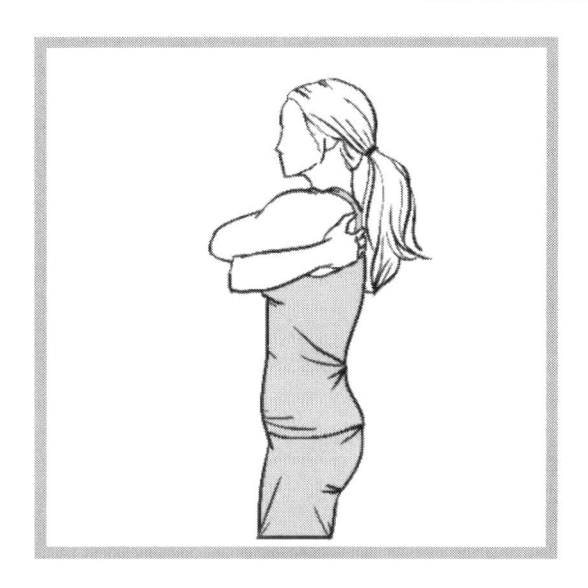

1. Self-hug Stretch

- Relax your shoulders. Take each of your hands and grab the opposite shoulder.
- Your arms should be one on top of the other and create a V shape on your chest. Your hands should be placed more to the side of the shoulder, not on top.
- Drop your shoulders down as far as you can get them while still keeping your eyes in front of you. Tuck your chin in.
- Let your chin drop towards your chest so that you will be moving your eyes towards the ground. Your chin should still be tucked.

- You should feel the stretch in the middle-upper part of your back. As soon as you feel the stretch, hold it for five breaths. Your shoulders should not be moving when you breathe.

This stretch lengthens the upper part of your back. If your back is very straight, this could compromise how your neck mechanics work; this stretch will loosen this up by introducing a slight forward arch. Loosened back and neck will reduce the risk of injury when you are lifting heavyweights.

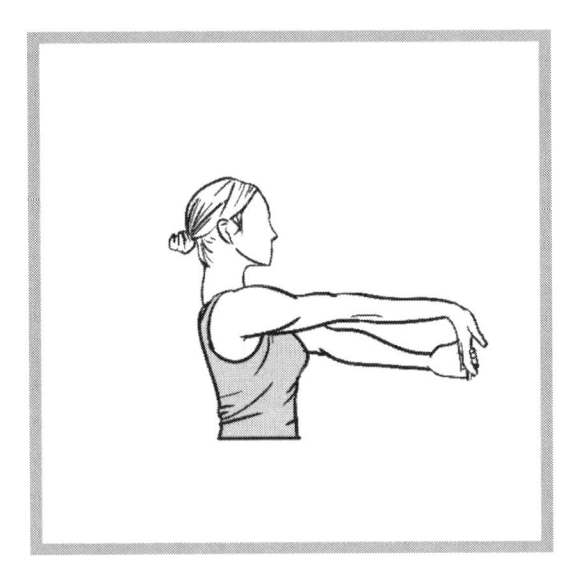

2. Forearm Stretch

- Stretch your arms out straight in front of you.

USE IT OR LOSE IT

- Flip your wrist up so that your fingers are pointing to the ceiling.
- Take one of your hands and pull back the fingers of the other hand.
- You should feel this stretch both in your wrist and the inner part of your forearm.
- Hold for 30 seconds.
- Next, flip your wrist downwards and curl your fingers in.
- With the other hand, pull the curled hand towards you.
- You will feel the stretch running up the back of the forearm.
- Hold for 30 seconds.
- Repeat this stretch three times each on both sides.

Stretching your forearms can often be overlooked, but this stretch stretches both the forearm and the fingers. You need your forearms to lift and your finger flexon to grip. After a long day of not using the forearm muscles, they become tight and shrink. Most jobs do not require the use of the forearm muscle, so it is our responsibility to make sure this muscle is engaged, so it has good mobility.

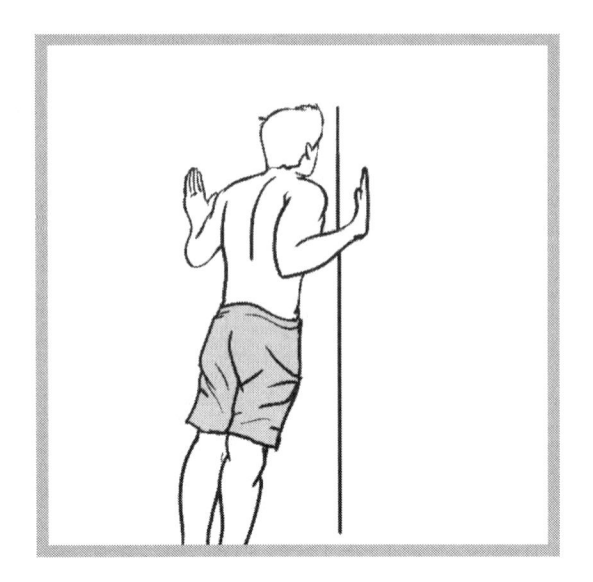

3. Corner Pec Stretch

- Stand a few feet away from the corner of a wall. You will have to adjust how far you stand, depending on your height and the length of your arms.
- Place your palms on either side of the wall at shoulder level.
- Breathe in, and then as you exhale, engage your core and pull them into your back, press your chest into the wall by leaning into it with your whole body.
- Your body should not be bending to accommodate

this move. Hold for 30 seconds and repeat three to five times.

- Holding this position results in the chest muscles lengthening.

This stretch targets the pectoralis minor, which is vital in the posture of your upper body. Tight pecs may lead to a hunched back because when they have not been stretched enough, they shrink and pull your shoulders in. It is vital to have good posture when working out and in general. You will not be able to get the best out of your upper body workouts if you do not address posture issues, it is better to prevent this then try and fix it when you already have it.

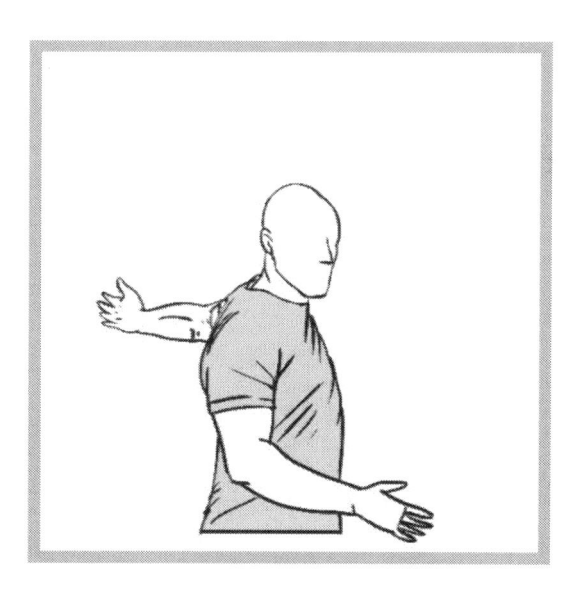

4. Big Turn Back Stretch

- Face a wall and stand as close to it as possible.
- Place your right arm flat against the wall with your palm on the wall. Your arm should be perpendicular to your body and completely straight against the wall.
- Slowly start rotating your torso to the left, leaving your arm stuck against the wall.
- Stop when you feel the stretch in your shoulder and chest. You can continue to deepen the stretch slowly, if you would like more of a stretch, make sure you do not take it too far.
- Hold for about 30 seconds and repeat on the other side.

This stretch helps open up your chest, stretch out your biceps, and loosen up your shoulders. It also has a positive effect on your posture. You will be using all of these muscles for lifting, pressing, and any other upper body workouts.

USE IT OR LOSE IT

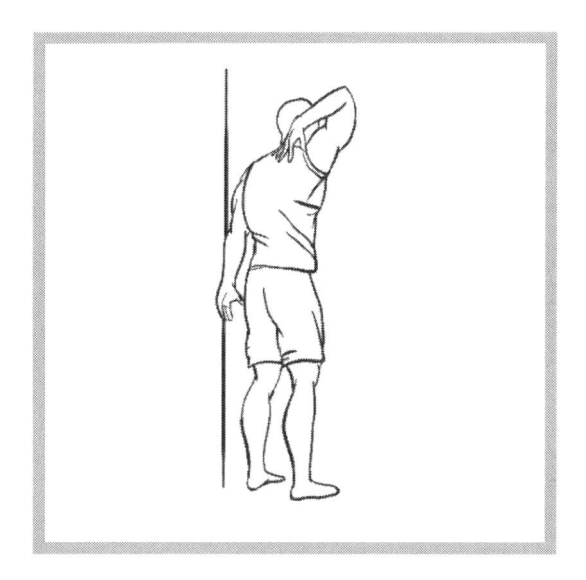

5. Wall Triceps Stretch

- Bend your left arm at the elbow and place the elbow on the wall, slide it up so that it is above your head. Your hand should be behind you, at the center of your back.
- Take your right hand and grab your left wrist.
- Lean into the wall and feel the stretch.
- Hold for 30 seconds and repeat on the other side.

The triceps are used to help move and extend the elbow, and it also plays a role in keeping the shoulder stable. Your whole arm and shoulders will loosen up and be more mobile if you use this stretch.

Most of us have experienced a spine that clicks at some point, the clicking or popping has to do with the general muscle and joint function. There is usually nothing wrong with cracking your back, but it can indicate that you have not been working on or stretching your spine enough. The spine holds up your entire upper body, so we want it to be mobile and functioning correctly. Doing a stretch is a good way of keeping the spine supple, and if done regularly, will hold less tension.

Thoracic Routine

The thoracic region is the region from below your shoulders to above your hips, your abdominal area. This region contains twelve vertebrae and your ribs; all your vital organs are found in this part of the body.

When you work out, your muscles heal and shorten; this happens especially when you sleep. Shortened muscles mean stiff muscles, and this can negatively impact your next workout. To help ease this and help you be in a better position for your next workout, you need to stretch out the thoracic region.

USE IT OR LOSE IT

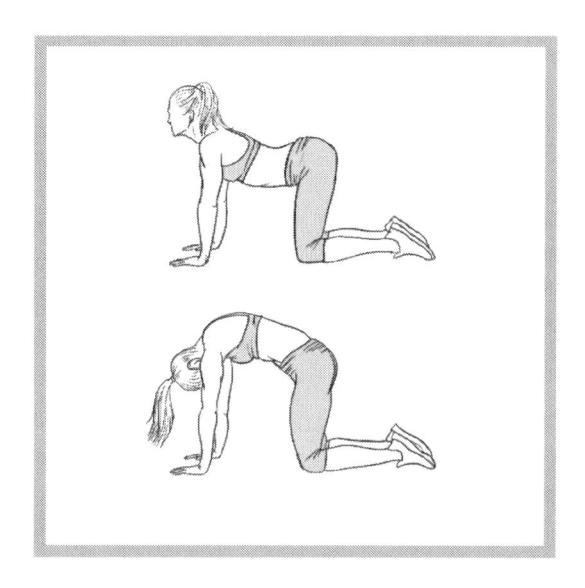

1. Cat-Cow

- Follow the instructions for the Cat-Cow Stretch under the Back and Torso routine in chapter 2.

This stretch has been known to improve balance significantly, and it engages all the vertebrae. It engages the tailbone to activate the root movement of the spine; this allows the spine to bend more freely. When your spine is more flexible and has a higher mobility, it will reduce your risk of injuries for many different workouts.

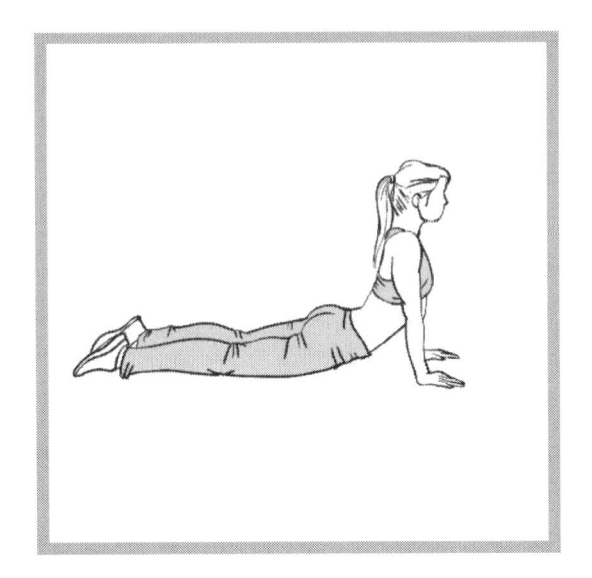

2. The Cobra

- Follow the instructions for the Cobra Stretch under the Back and Torso routine in chapter 2.

The cobra is a spinal stretch that will strengthen your spine. It is also suitable for stretching out the chest, shoulder, and abdomen. Daily activities can impact your spine and spine health, sitting at a desk or even carrying a child causes our spine to bend forward. This can hinder us in many areas, including our fitness, this stretch helps counteract some of the effects of our daily lives.

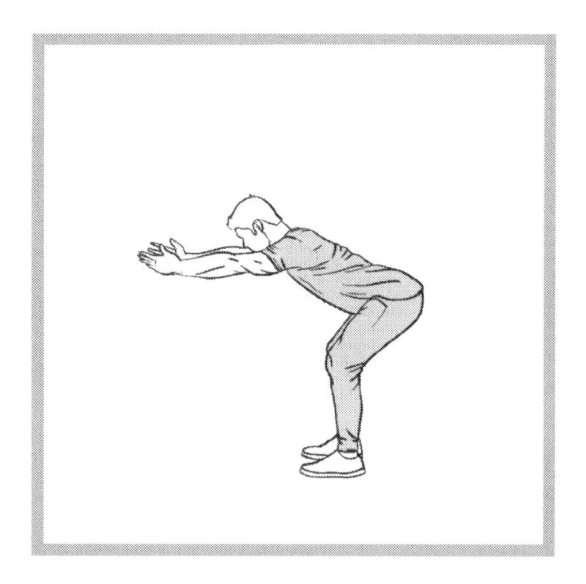

3. The Hip Hinge

- Follow the instructions for the hip hinge under the Back and Torso routine in chapter 2.

Bending is part of our general lives, so we need to have a strong core and lower spinal area. This is also important when it comes to strength training, deadlifts, kettlebell swings, and many other exercises that require you to have a strong lower back and core. This stretch strengthens your spine and core so that you have mobility in these areas.

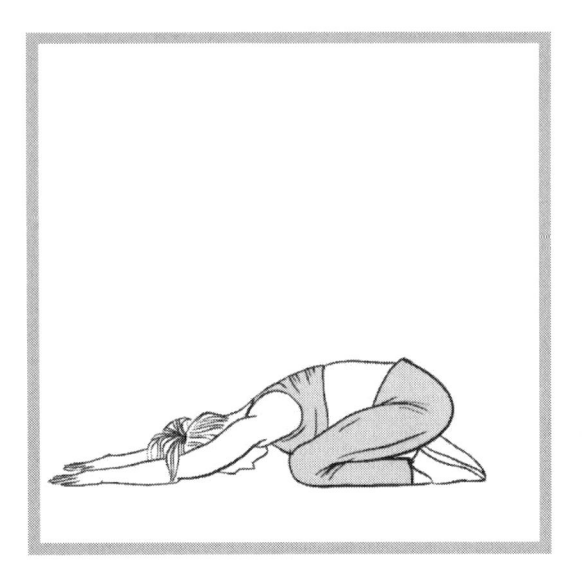

4. Child's Pose

- Follow the instructions for the Child's Pose under the Neck, Shoulder, and Chest routine in chapter 2.

Child's pose is incredibly versatile in terms of what body parts it stretches out. It helps with stabilizing the spine and opening up the chest and hips. We tend to have compression in our lower backs because we push our extra weight there instead of engaging our abdominal muscles. This pose helps us release that compression and can make us more conscious of engaging our core.

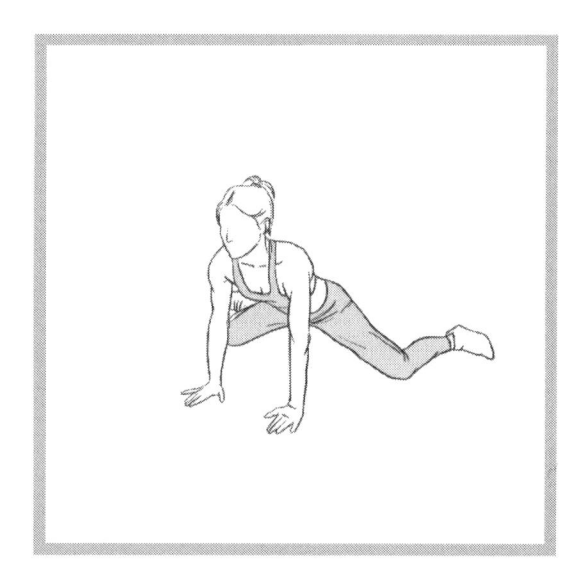

5. The Frog Stretch

- Get down on your hands and knees.
- Turn your feet inwards so that the inner part of the foot is on the floor, and slide your knees apart. They should be wider than your shoulders.
- Drop your hips towards your feet.
- If you can get down onto your forearms instead of on your hands, this will give you a deeper stretch.
- Hold for 30 seconds to 2 minutes.

This stretch works on your groin and adductors, but it also targets your core, which is why it is in this routine. If you have done any kind of exercise or are an athlete of any kind, you will know how important the core is to almost anything you do. Your core muscles are where most of your strength comes from, so having a flexible and robust core will improve your ability in any exercise.

Lower Back and Hips

Building up your flexibility, mobility, and strength in your lower back and hips is the best way to prevent injuries in these areas. A lower back and hip injuries are amongst the most common in the fitness world. Not only is preventing injury important, but strengthening this area helps you get a better lower body workout and upper body workout. This area sits in the middle of your body, and it tends to carry a lot of weight and pressure from exercise and daily activity. Follow this routine to strengthen your lower back and hips.

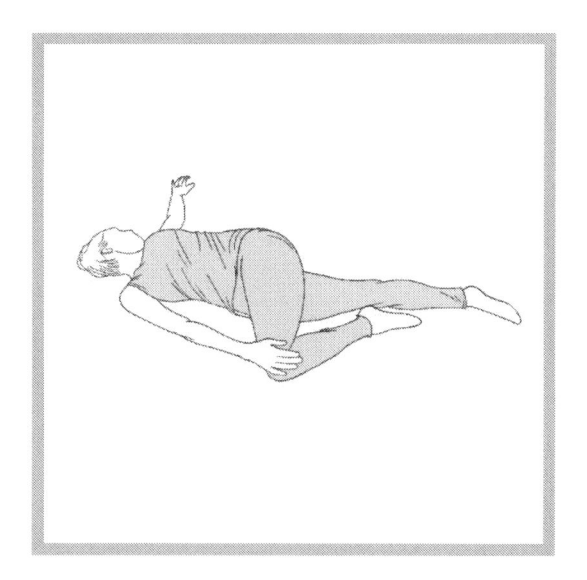

1. Supine Spinal Stretch

- Lay down on your back and bring your right knee up to your chest.
- Take your left arm and bring your right knee down to cross the body and land on the left side.
- Stretch out your right arm to the side and turn your head to look at it.
- Hold for 30 seconds and repeat on the other side.

This move helps stretch out your spine, lower back, and it opens up your chest, moving the lower body in a way that it usually doesn't target joints and muscles that are often neglected.

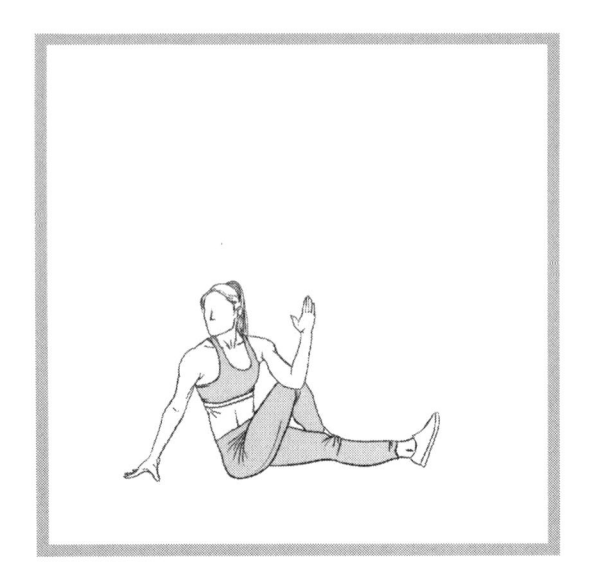

2. Seated Piriformis Stretch

- Sit on the edge of a chair with your back straight.
- Take your left leg and place the ankle on top of your right thigh. Flex the foot and let it be parallel to the floor.
- Pin down your leg by placing your hand on the ankle and the other hand on the thigh.
- Lean forward and bring your chest into your shin. Go as far as you can to deepen the stretch.
- Keep your back straight at all times.
- Hold for 30 seconds to 2 minutes and repeat on the other side.

This stretch will target the piriformis, glute, and outer hip joints and muscles. These muscles and joints are all important in the movement of the lower body. You will be using them whether you are performing strength training or doing athletic training.

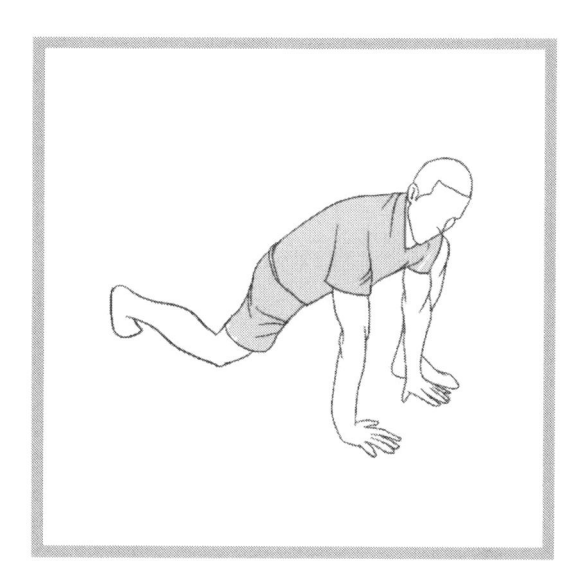

3. The Knight Stretch

- Follow the instructions for the Knight Stretch under the Knees and Thighs routine in chapter 2.

The knight stretch opens up your hips and stretches out your leg muscles; it also stretches your spine and opens up your chest. Stretches like these show you how one move can affect so many different parts of the body. It also shows how connected your body is and why mind-body balance is important.

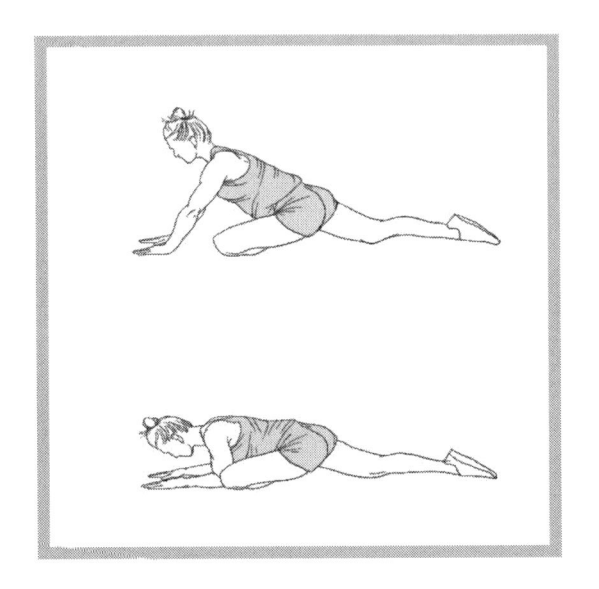

4. Pigeon Pose

- Follow the instructions for the Pigeon Pose under the Hips and Glutes routine in chapter 2.

When you have tight hip flexors, it pulls your pelvis forward, and this has some negative effects on your lower back. Your lower back might have an exaggerated arch, and what this means is that in certain positions or moves, you will feel pain. Loosening up those hip flexors with this stretch will help get a healthier back arch and give you more freedom when you are exercising.

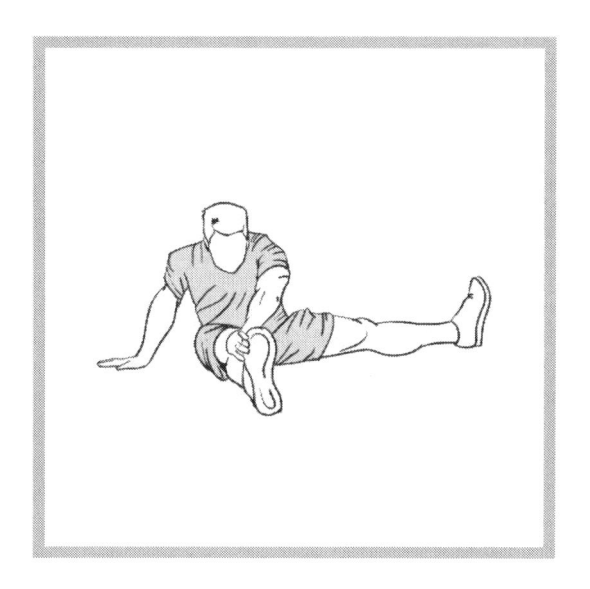

5. The V-Sit

- Sit on the floor with your back straight and your legs open as far apart as you can get them.
- Lean over with your whole body to try and reach your foot. You may not be able to grab your foot; in this case, grab your shin or thigh. Push down into your leg until you feel the stretch in your hamstring.
- Hold for 30 seconds and repeat on the other side.

This stretch will help you to measure the flexibility you have in your hamstrings and your lower back. Doing this stretch will allow you to have a wider range of motion in your hips and a stronger lower back.

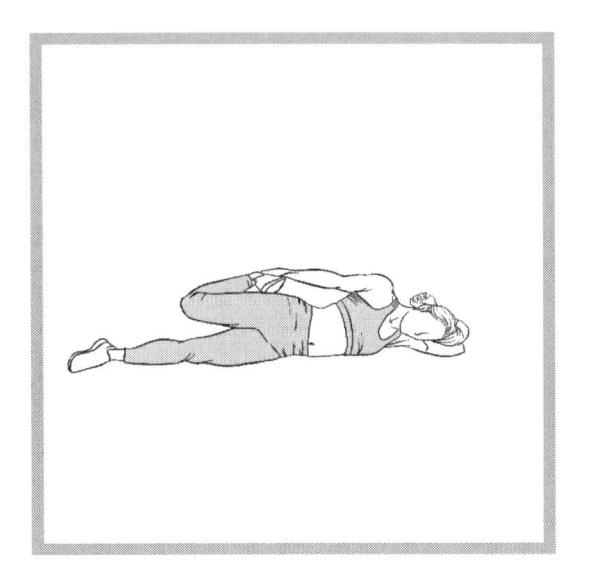

Lower Body

1. Quad Stretch

- Follow the instructions for the Quad Stretch under the Knees and Thighs routine in chapter 2.

This stretch works on not only the quads but also the hips, knee, and other muscles in the leg. This is especially good for strengthening and stretching your legs in preparation for intense lower-body movements. Cyclists, runners, and people who do yoga all look to this stretch to prepare them for their exercise and help them cool down afterward.

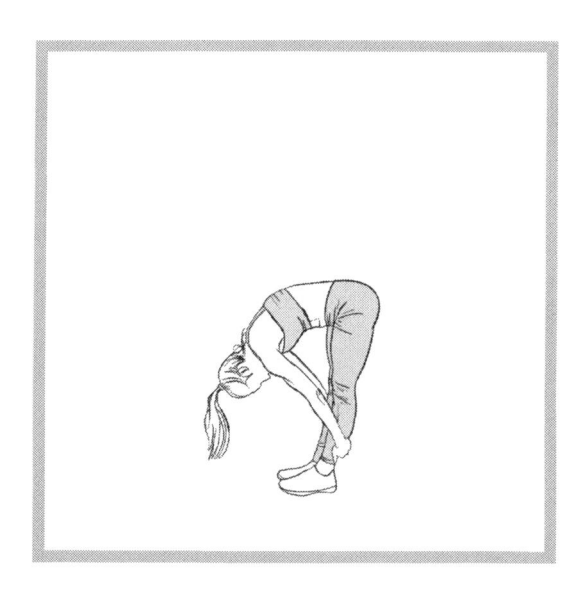

2. Hamstring Stretch

- Sit down on the ground with your legs straight out in front of you and your back straight.
- Breathe in and fold your body over your thighs, reach for your feet. If you cannot reach your feet, then go as far as you can until you feel the stretch in your hamstrings.
- If you want more of a stretch, you can flex your feet.

- Hold for 30 seconds, come back up and shake out your legs. Repeat three times.

Hamstring stretches help loosen up the hamstring, and as a result, this gives your body more support. A stringer hamstring will also offer your knees more support when running and performing other exercises.

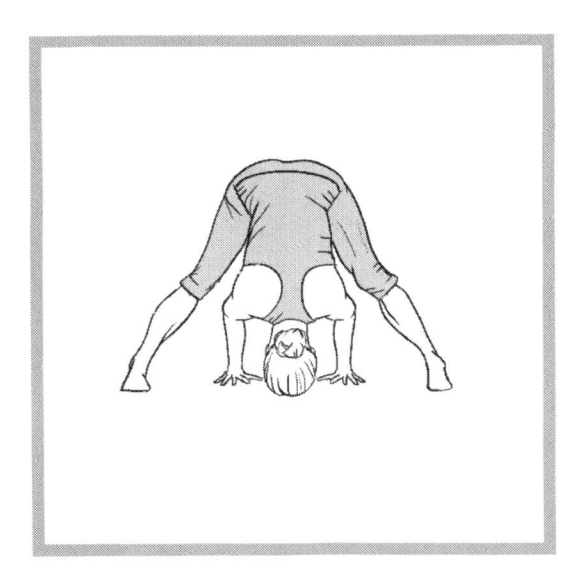

3. Standing Forward Fold

- Stand up with your back straight and feet apart.
- Bend at your hips and bring your body as close to your thighs as you can. Try and keep your knees straight as your reach for the floor with your

fingertips. If this is not possible, then reach for your ankles or calves.
- Try and move closer to your thighs with every exhale.
- Hold for 30 seconds to 1 minute.

This stretch will help lengthen the hamstrings and strengthen the knees and thighs. You might also feel something in your calves and hips; this is a stretch that works out most of your lower body.

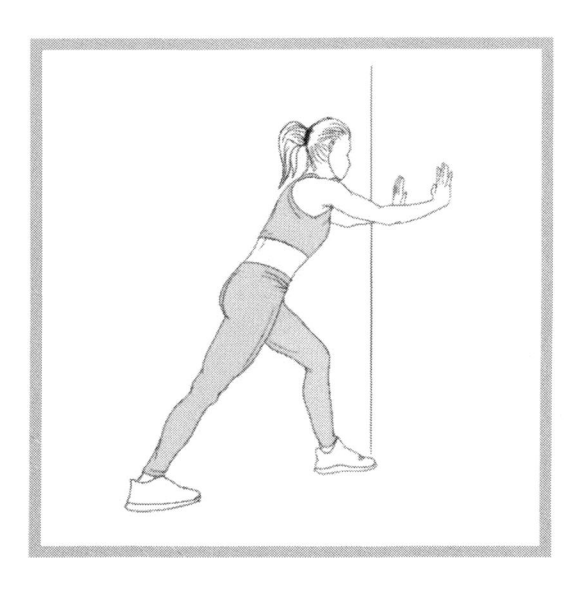

4. Wall Calf Stretch

- Stand a few feet away from a wall.

- Step forward with one leg and leave the other behind. Both feet should be facing forward.
- Hold your hands up against the wall.
- Bend the knee closest to the wall and keep the other leg straight.
- Lean into the wall with your body. Keep both feet planted on the ground. You should feel the stretch in the calf of your back leg.
- Hold for 30 seconds to 1 minute and repeat on the other side.

This stretch will work out your calf but also your Achilles tendon. This means that there will be a wider range of motion, and your lower leg and ankles will be strengthened.

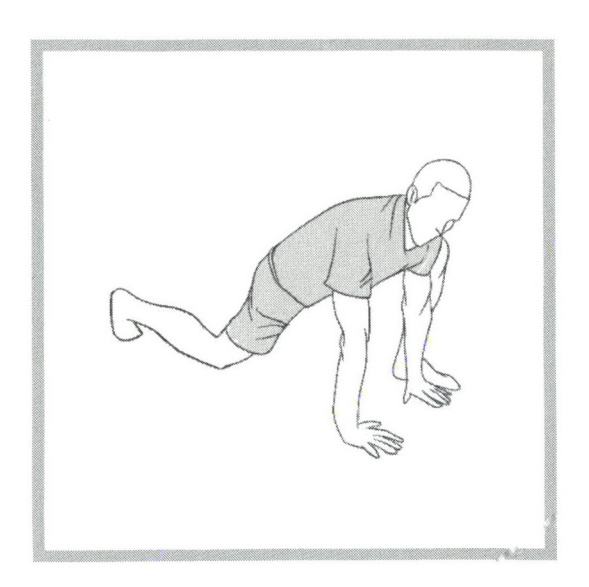

5. The Knight Stretch

- Follow the instructions for the Knight Stretch under the Knees and Thighs routine in chapter 2.

Also, see notes under the lower back and hips routine in this chapter.

THE COOL DOWN: THE ROUTINE TO KEEP YOU, YOUNG

Stretching has so many benefits, not only for your body but also for your mind and your overall well-being. It is a brilliant way to help with injuries and enhance workouts, but we cannot forget the other benefits that come along with it. In general, having excellent flexibility will add to your life, and being more mindful of your stretching can increase your quality of life to a level you would not expect.

THE ROUTINE

Before we jump into the routine, let's focus on meditation and breathing, which are yoga practices, but they extend further than that. These are essential aspects of stretching and improve the way you feel when you are done with the routine and throughout the rest of the day. They help us connect with our bodies and increase how effective our stretches can be.

The importance of yoga is that it does not focus just on the physical body but on the mind as well. What goes on in our mind can affect our bodies, that is why it is so important to be mindful and be able to take control of our thoughts. This is where meditation comes in; meditation helps get the mind-body balance right. It helps us to focus our minds on what is going on in our body, and we can respond to this effectively. Our mind and body are not separate entities, but instead, they work together. This, in turn, will help with everyday movements and control of your emotions, which believe it or not have a huge effect on the pain we feel in our body too. The power to be in control of your mind and your body will lead to a more fulfilling life. This will also be reflected in the response of your body.

Breathing, as we know, is important in general life, but it is essential in stretching. When we focus on breathing, we start focusing on our bodies; this can lead to a lower risk of injury. Breathing will increase our oxygen intake; our muscles need the oxygen to run at their best. Be mindful of when you exhale and inhale, this can also be a tool to help deepen your stretches and reduce the stress that causes knots and tension.

Now let's get into the stretching routine. This routine is excellent for increasing flexibility in your whole body; it was developed by Winderl (2020). Paired with the breathing and meditation techniques we have just spoken about, it is a winning combination for a full mind and body routine.

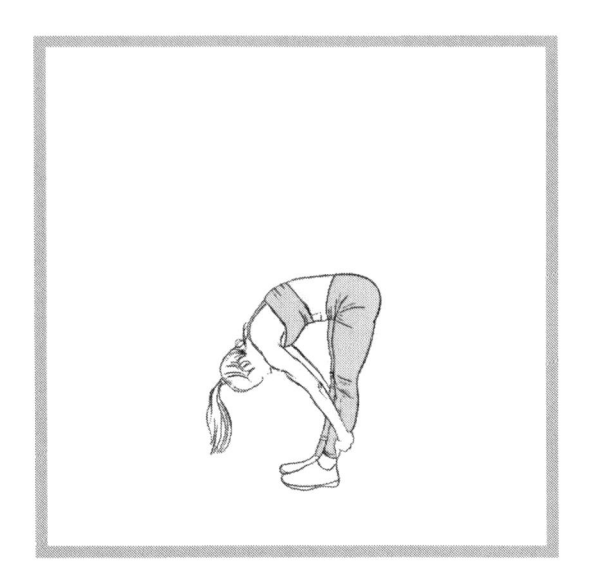

1. Standing Hamstring Stretch

- Start by standing up straight with your feet aligned with your hips.
- Breathe in and fold your body over at the hips, grab the back of your legs at the lowest point you can get it.
- Your upper body should be relaxed.

- Hold for 45 seconds - 2 minutes.

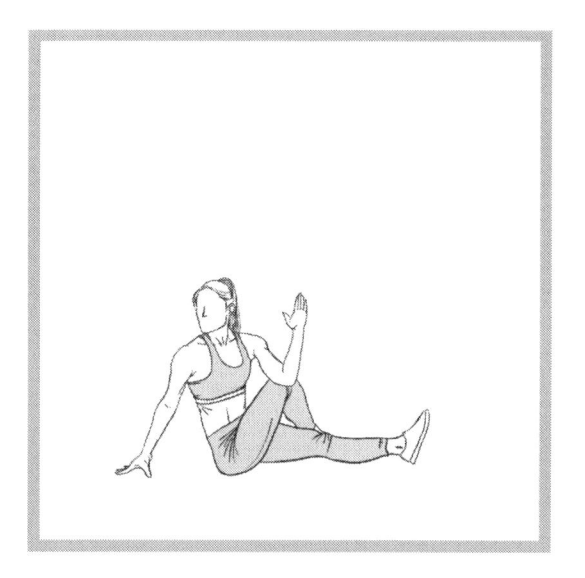

2. Piriformis Stretch

- Follow the instructions for the Piriformis Stretch under the Back and Torso routine in chapter 2.

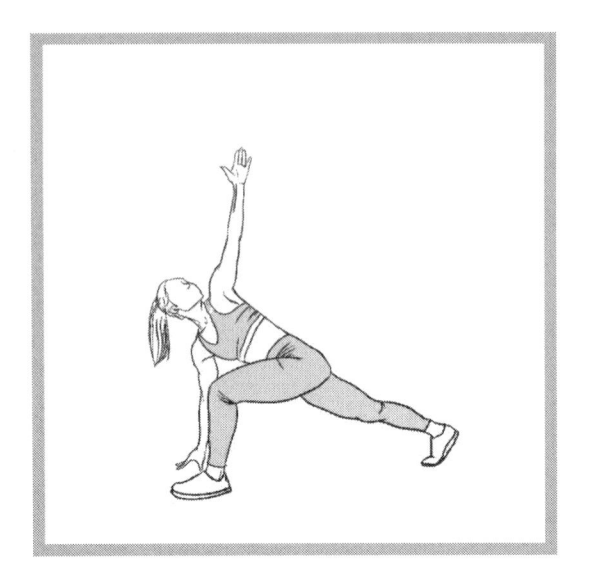

3. Lunge With Spinal Twist

- Follow the instructions for the Lunge With Spinal Twist stretch under the Hips and Glutes routine in chapter 2.

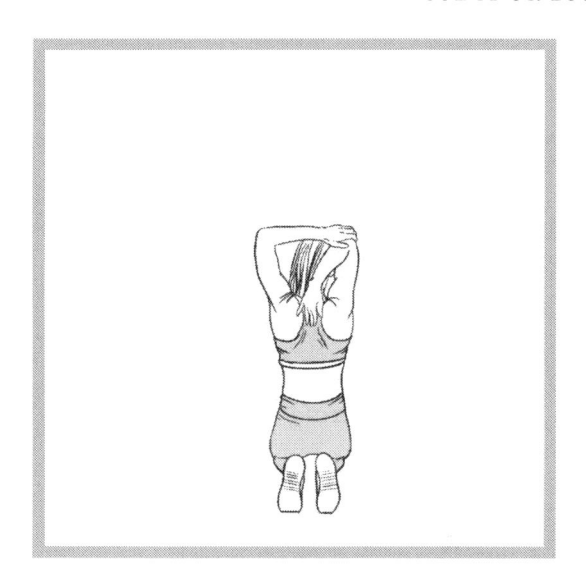

4. Triceps Stretch

- You may stand, kneel, or sit for this stretch.
- Extend your arms above you.
- Bend your arms at the elbow, and touch the center of the top of your back with your hand.
- With your other hand, reach over and grab and pull down gently on the elbow of the bent arm.
- Hold for 30 seconds, repeat on the other side.

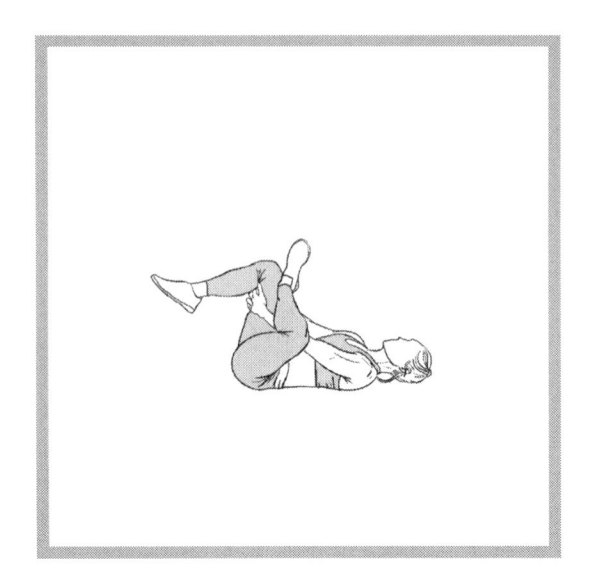

5. Lying Figure 4 Stretch

- Follow the instructions for the Lying Figure 4 Stretch under the Hips and Glutes routine in chapter 2.

USE IT OR LOSE IT

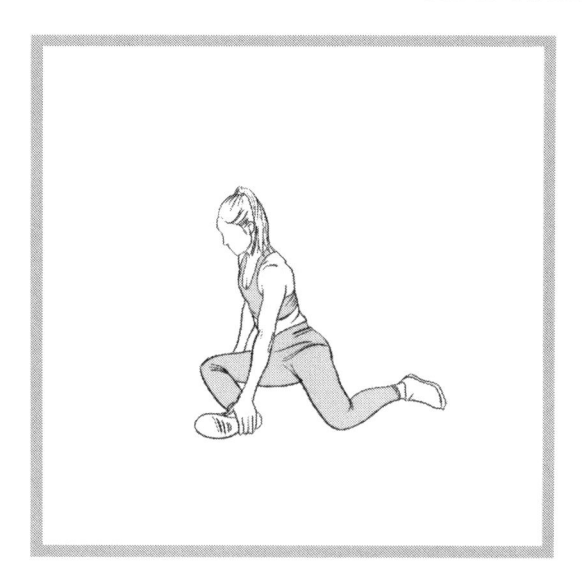

6. 90/90 Stretch

- Follow the instructions for the 90/90 Stretch under the Hips and Glutes routine in chapter 2.

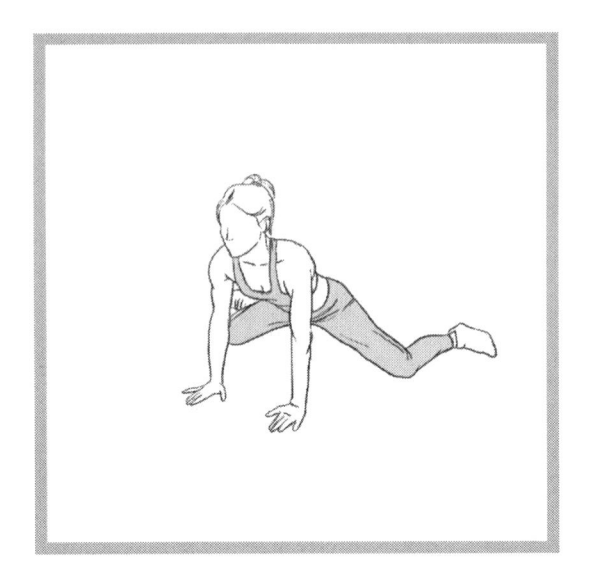

7. The Frog Stretch

- Follow the instructions for the Frog Stretch under the Thoracic routine in chapter 4.

USE IT OR LOSE IT

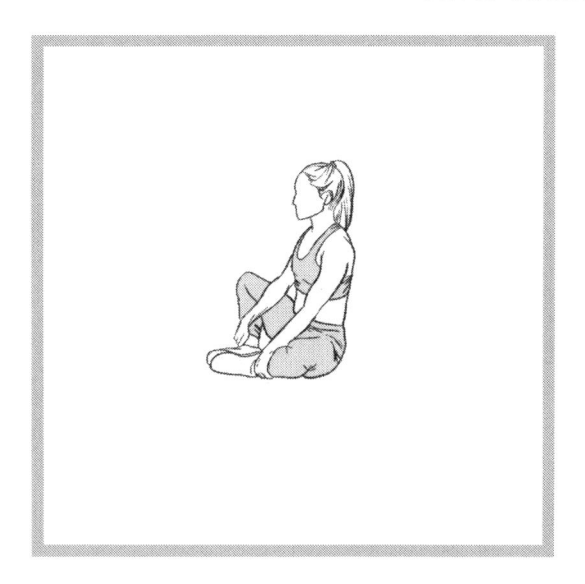

8. Butterfly Stretch

- Sit on the floor with the bottoms of your feet touching.
- Lean over and try to get your head as close to the floor as possible. Push down on your knees with your elbows.
- The closer your feet are to you, the deeper the stretch will be.
- Hold for 30 seconds to 2 minutes.

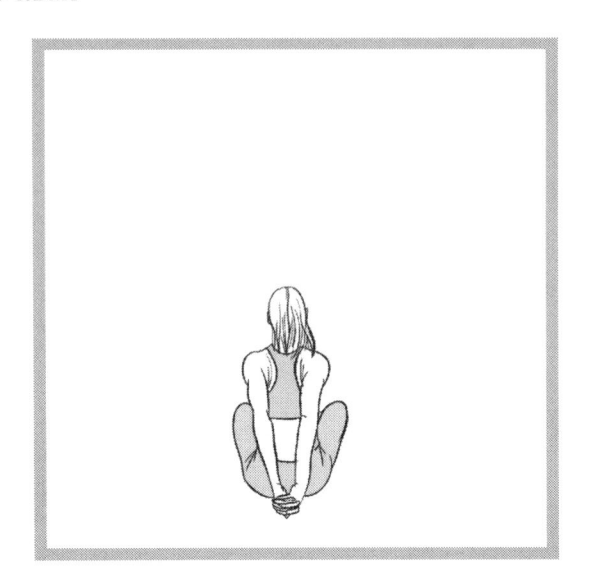

9. Seated Shoulder Squeeze

- Sit down on the ground, bend your knees and have your feet flat on the ground.
- Interlock your fingers behind you.
- Straighten out your arms; you will feel your shoulder blades pulling together.
- Hold for 3 seconds—repeat between five and ten times.

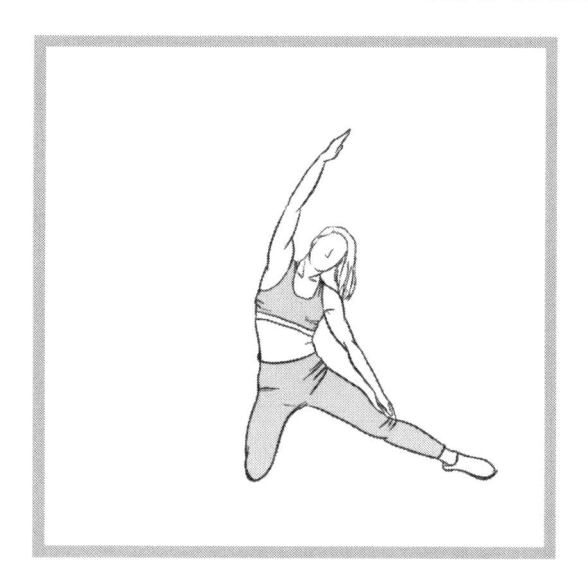

10. Side Bend Stretch

- Kneel on the ground. Keep your back straight.
- Straighten out your right leg to the side.
- Place your right arm on your right leg and lift your left arm in the air.
- Lean your body and arm over to the right.
- Your hips should be facing straight in front of you and your right leg perpendicular to your body.
- Hold between 30 seconds and 2 minutes.

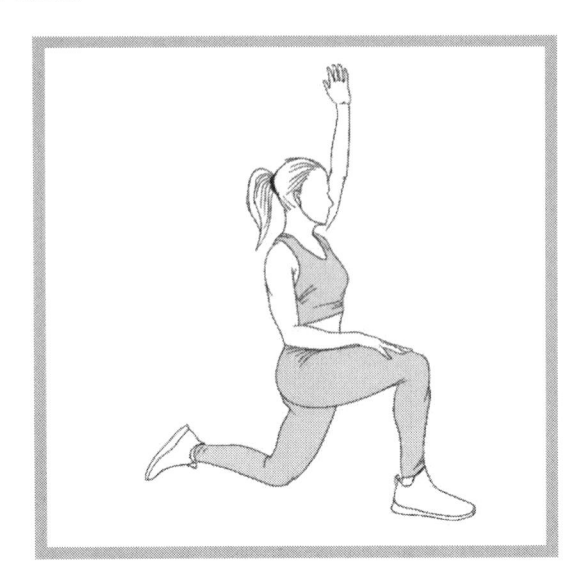

11. Lunging Hip Flexor Stretch

- Kneel on one knee.
- Lean into the leg that is in front of you with your hips.
- If you squeeze your butt, it will give you more of a stretch.
- Hold between 30 seconds and 2 minutes. Repeat on the other side.

USE IT OR LOSE IT

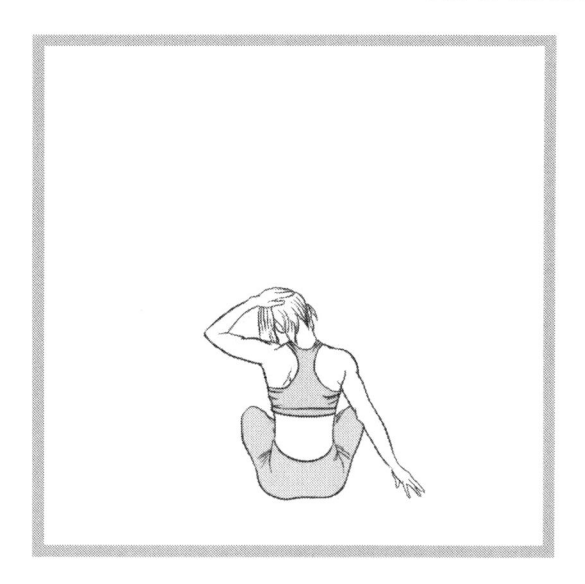

12. Seated Neck Release

- Sit or stand with your back straight.
- Move your right ear towards your right shoulder.
- Take your right hand and slowly pull your head closer to your shoulder.
- Hold between 30 seconds and 2 minutes.

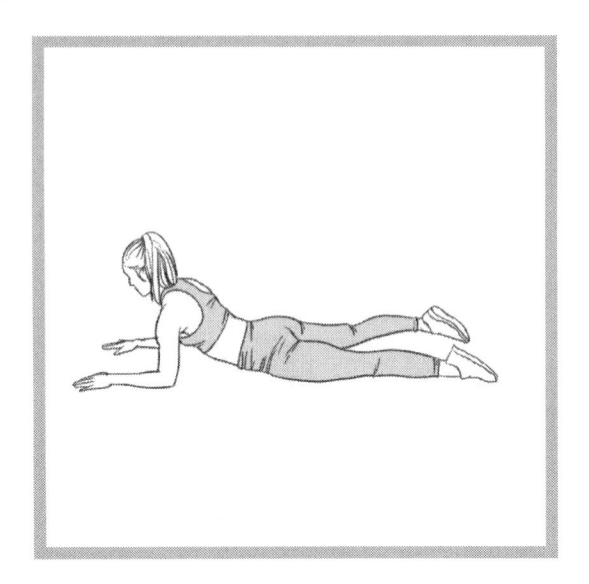

13. Sphinx Pose

- Follow the instructions for the Sphinx Pose under the Back and Torso routine in chapter 2.

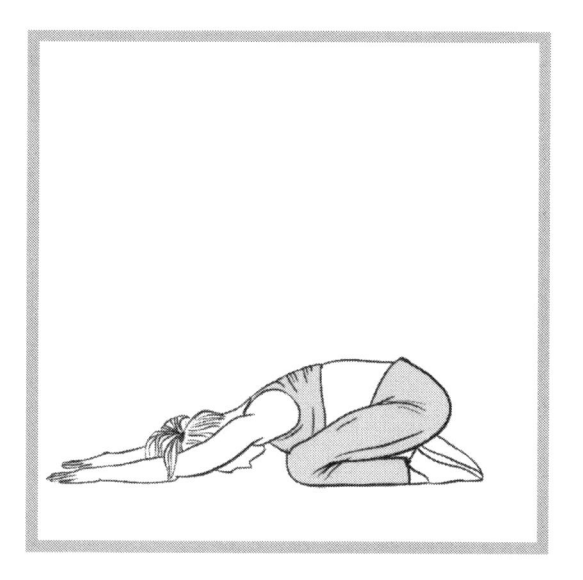

14. Child's Pose

- Follow the instructions for the Child's Pose under the Neck, Shoulder, and Chest routine in chapter 2.

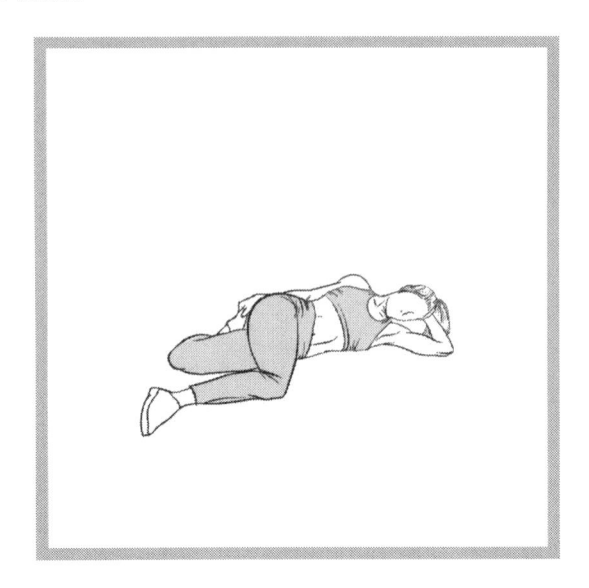

15. Pretzel Stretch

- Lay on the ground flat on your right side. Rest your head on your arm.
- Bend your left leg and bring it up as close to your body as possible.
- Bend your right leg back and grab it with your free arm, pull it up as close to your butt as possible.
- Slowly bring your left shoulder towards the ground, while keeping your torso straight.
- Hold between 30 seconds and 2 minutes. Repeat on the other side.

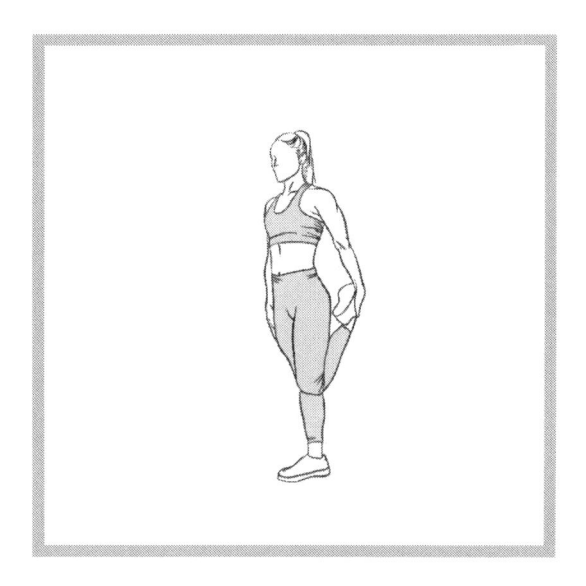

16. Standing Quad Stretch

- Stand up with your back straight and feet together.
- Bend one of your knees back and grab your foot with your hand. Pull the foot towards your butt.
- Do not let your knees separate.
- Squeeze your butt for more of a stretch.
- Hold between 30 seconds and 2 minutes.
- Repeat on the other side.

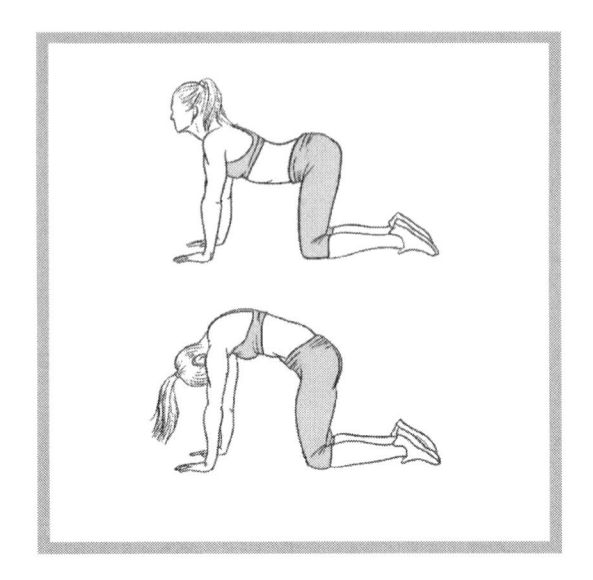

17. Cat-Cow Stretch

- Follow the instructions for the Cat-Cow Stretch under the Back and Torso routine in chapter 2.

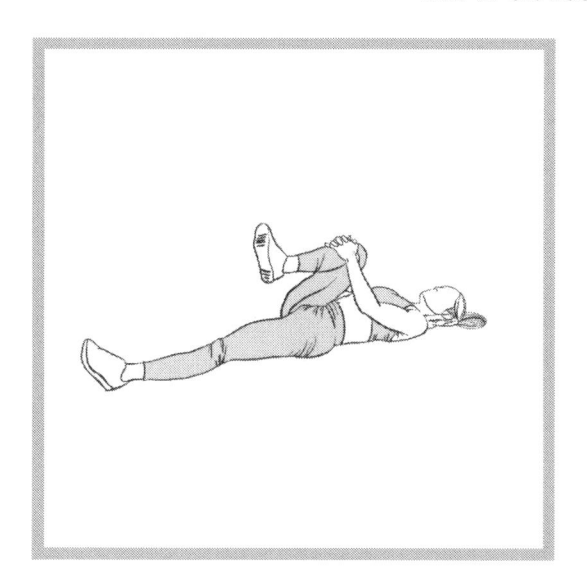

18. Knees to Chest

- Lay down on the ground with your back on the floor.
- Bring your knees up towards your chest.
- Hold onto your shins with your hands and pull them into you.
- Don't allow your lower back to lift off the floor.
- Hold between 30 seconds and 2 minutes.

LIVE A HEALTHY LIFESTYLE

No part of your body runs on its own. Everything is connected and works together for the good or the bad of the entire body and mind. That is why it would not be right to just talk about stretching without mentioning some other aspects that work with stretching to keep you healthy and happy.

We must never forget that no matter how much stretching and exercise we do, if we do not feed ourselves the right nutrition, it might all be in vain. What you eat and how your body performs work side by side. This is why we need to pay attention to what we are putting in our bodies; it can either fuel us or zap our energy. Stick to foods that are high in nutrients, pick whole foods, and always try and incorporate fruits and vegetables into your meals wherever you can. You will feel the difference in your body, in your mind, and your energy levels. Vitamin B is essential within body processes such as energy production.

Sleep is also an important part of a healthy lifestyle. Most people overlook sleep, but it is what will give us energy for the next day. When we sleep, our body repairs itself, and our mind resets itself to prepare for the next day. When we get too little sleep or low quality sleep, we rob our bodies of the opportunity to do this, and before we even get a chance to decide how the day is going to go, we are already on the back foot. If you sleep well, your body will function better; you will be sharper and make better decisions throughout the day. Sleep is one of the main issues I encounter when training clients, and before you work on your fitness and flexibility, getting your sleep right is hugely important.

Give biohacking a try; it can help you discover more about yourself. What your body likes and doesn't like, and how it responds to different patterns and foods. Biohacking is making small changes to your life and lifestyle so that you can see changes in your health and well-being (Jewell, 2019). Much of biohacking is trial and error, or some may describe it as split-testing, but it can help you get a better understanding of your specific body. You could try a diet where you remove one thing and then slowly reintroduce it and see how it makes you feel, or try adding caffeine to your diet as a productivity and energy booster. Try going to bed at different times or having a different bedtime routine and take note of how it affects your sleep. The good thing about biohacking is that you might uncover a secret to a better life that you didn't know before.

When you have a healthy lifestyle, it causes a ripple effect in your life that flows into many areas. Think about it; when you are healthy, you have positive inputs that will respond with positive outputs and responses. You will notice your body thanking you through less pain and your mind thanking you through more emotional control and fewer swings. It affects the way you think because you are more positive and positivity breeds opportunity. You will be more motivated to live better and give more. Other people want to be around happy people. This will vastly improve your relationships and help you to create new ones, stronger ones. Let's not forget how stretching can boost your mood as well; when we stretch, our body releases endorphins, which give us a high and lift our mood. This feeling can last many hours after you have finished stretching and can translate into how you handle situations and people around you.

At the core of this healthy lifestyle is a mind-body balance. We need to have this because it is so important to be healthy all around and not just in one aspect; if we focus too much on one thing, we will not be steady, and it won't be long before we crumble under the pressure of whatever comes our way. Health is made up of pillars of mind and body, and we need to make sure both of them are strong.

It's all well and good to say that you need this balance, but the big question is how to get it. There are actually quite a few things you can do in your life to help you get to a state of overall wellness. Get up and get moving. Sitting down for too long can have negative effects on your body and mind. Aim for 15 minutes of heart elevating activity every day. Do something that feeds your soul, ask yourself where your passion lies, and find a way to integrate that into your life. Treat everyone with kindness, give back, and take the time to slow down and be a part of the world around you and

USE IT OR LOSE IT

practice gratification. One of the most important ones is to remember to laugh, those same endorphins that are released when you stretch are released when you laugh. These are only a few of the ways you can move towards a mind-body balance, and anything that brings you joy and peace can be added to this list.

There are many facets to health, so remember to explore and pay attention to all of them. Balance is achievable if you take the right steps towards it. It isn't a foreign or make-believe concept but rather something available to all of us. It is your life and your body, and you want to live it the best you can, so whatever that is, make every decision from now in aid of moving in that direction.

<u>FREE</u> WORKOUT PLANNER & KILLER CORE WORKOUT

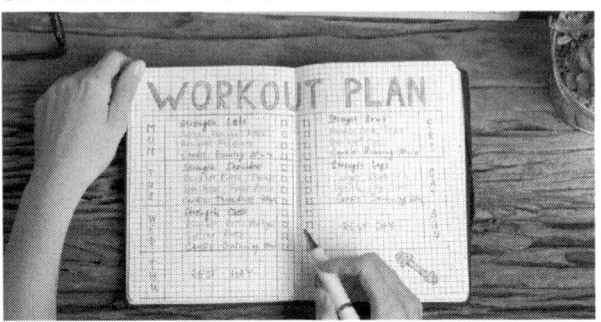

Want to make sure you reach your fitness goals?....you won't without tracking your progress! and did you know most exercises depend on a strong core for results?

1. Get your FREE perfect workout planner.
2. Get my FREE killer core workout so you reach your goals faster
3. Simply print off or download onto your device
4. And feel amazing as you watch your progress skyrocket

to receive just type in the following link :).......

https://fitnessmilo.activehosted.com/f/1

YOUR MISSION SHOULD YOU CHOOSE TO ACCEPT IT…….

I need your help; I am new to publishing and working my socks off day and night to try and bring you the best content in my books.

So, your mission from me is that if you enjoyed the book, leave me a quick and honest review. So we can get my books seen by more people and let them know the quality of my books, this is top secret information and we are running out of time.

P.S. if you did not enjoy the book, instead of leaving a negative review, please contact me letting me know why you did not like the content, and I will do my best to address your concerns

Thank you :)

CONCLUSION

Stiffness and lack of mobility is something that many people just silently suffer from purely because they don't know what to do or where to turn to for help. Luckily that does not have to be your story. The stretches and routines in this book have covered every part of the body that no matter where your problem areas are, you are now equipped to handle them head-on.

Taking what you have learned and letting these stretches guide you will be the deciding factor of whether your body and mind reach its full potential. The body is a beautiful thing; it is the case in which our lives are held, so we should want to take care of it. There is no better way to take care of our body than to give it back its flexibility and full range of motion that has been taken away by sedentary lifestyles or unfortunate circumstances.

CONCLUSION

Whether you want to take the stretches and create your routine or have a specific goal in mind like getting past an injury that is slowing you down, these stretches will help you. As we have discussed, stretching can also help you optimize your workouts, so this is not just for beginners; in fact, you can start at any level and improve wherever you are. Stretching is beneficial to whoever gives it a shot and wants to see what their bodies can do.

Stretching is not only about improving your body and the physical aspects of your life, but it is about adding something to your routine that will help you live a better overall life. The ripple effect of having a good stretching routine implemented in your life is incredible. From having more mobility and freedom to just being in a better mood and having a clearer mind, these are all available to you if you are willing to put in a bit of effort to see your life change for the better.

Give it a shot, and you will not regret it. The fantastic thing is that you do not have to wait months to reap the benefits stretching offers. Your body will start feeling better quicker than you expect, and your emotions and morality will change and become healthier. That is the goal at the end of the day. We all want to be healthier in all aspects of our lives. Stay committed to the process, and your future self will be thanking you.

REFERENCES

AskDoctorJo. (2012, June 22). Shoulder Pain Treatment & Rehab Stretches - Ask Doctor Jo [Video File] Retrieved May 14, 2020, from https://www.youtube.com/watch?v=DJvQ3ZGWUfQ

AskDoctorJo. (2012, June 22). Back Pain Relief with Extension & Rotation Stretches - Ask Doctor Jo. [Video File] Retrieved May 14, 2020, from https://www.youtube.com/watch?v=wgPf9IJiW5s

AskDoctorJo. (2012, October 2012). Pulled Groin Pain Stretches - Ask Doctor Jo. [Video File] Retrieved May 14, 2020, from https://www.youtube.com/watch?v=22tWXwZ2DF8

AskDoctorJo. (2013, March 13). Quadriceps Stretches for Tight or Injured Quads - Ask Doctor Jo. [Video File]

REFERENCES

Retrieved May 14, 2020, from https://www.youtube.com/watch?v=BhQimqvU1tM

AskDoctorJo. (2013, March 17). Quadriceps Stretches for Tight or Injured Quads - Ask Doctor Jo Retrieved May 16, 2020, from https://www.youtube.com/watch?v=BhQimqvU1tM

AskDoctorJo. (2013, March 18). Achilles Tendon Stretches - Ask Doctor Jo. [Video File] Retrieved May 14, 2020, from https://www.youtube.com/watch?v=vU_FVahd4HI

AskDoctorJo. (2013, March 20). Hip Flexor Stretches & Exercises - Ask Doctor Jo. [Video File] Retrieved May 16, 2020, from https://www.youtube.com/watch?v=7bRaX6M2nr8

AskDoctorJo. (2013, July 4). Hip Pain & Knee Pain Exercises, Seated - Ask Doctor Jo. [Video File] Retrieved May 14, 2020, from https://www.youtube.com/watch?v=4z5W03XutXg

AskDoctorJo. (2016, May 23). Hamstring Strain Stretches & Exercises - Ask Doctor Jo. [Video File] Retrieved May 14, 2020, from https://www.youtube.com/watch?v=x5gunCRsSPU

AskDoctorJo. (2016, July 26). Hand Arthritis Stretches & Exercises - Ask Doctor Jo. [Video File] Retrieved May 16,

2020, from https://www.youtube.com/watch?v=tRnqF-AFFdw

AskDoctorJo. (2017, August 13). Gluteus Maximus (Glute) Strain Stretches & Exercises - Ask Doctor Jo. [Video File] Retrieved May 14, 2020, from https://www.youtube.com/watch?v=Y3T4IedBd4o&t=247s

AskDoctorJo. (2017, August 16). Wrist Tendonitis Treatment for Pain Relief - Ask Doctor Jo [Video File] Retrieved May 14, 2020, from https://www.youtube.com/watch?v=E7vibxI3yZY&t=665s

AskDoctorJo (2017, August 29). Calf Pain or Strain Stretches & Exercises - Ask Doctor Jo. [Video File] Retrieved May 14, 2020, from https://www.youtube.com/watch?v=XibsfBav_04&t=306s

AskDoctorJo (2017, September 13). 10 Best Rotator Cuff Pain Stretches - Ask Doctor Jo. [Video File] Retrieved May 14, 2020, from https://www.youtube.com/watch?v=hd5TY9c1dLE&t=420s

AskDoctorJo (2018, April 2). 5 Best Carpal Tunnel Syndrome Stretches & Exercises - Ask Doctor Jo [Video File] Retrieved May 16, 2020, from https://www.youtube.com/watch?v=Q5G916yCyF0

AskDoctorJo (2019, July 29). 7 Easy Carpal Tunnel

REFERENCES

Syndrome Treatments - Ask Doctor Jo. [Video File] Retrieved May 16, 2020 https://www.youtube.com/watch?v=FoKUWlKK_Vc

Axtell, B. (2018, February 26). 9 Foot Exercises to Try at Home. Retrieved May 14, 2020, from https://www.healthline.com/health/fitness-exercise/foot-exercises#marble-pickup

Bedosky, L. (2018, October 15). What's the Difference Between Mobility and Flexibility? | Fitness | MyFitnessPal. Retrieved May 11, 2020, from https://blog.myfitnesspal.com/whats-the-difference-between-mobility-and-flexibility/

Bodyfix, M.-. T. O. O. (2020, April 27). How do spiky massage balls work to relieve muscle tension? Retrieved May 13, 2020, from https://www.mybodyfix.co.nz/blog/how-do-spikey-massage-balls-work/

Cavaliere, J. (n.d.). 4 Stretches You Should Be Doing EVERY Morning! Retrieved May 17, 2020, from https://athleanx.com/articles/4-stretches-you-should-be-doing-every-morning

Cronkleton, E. (2020, May 4). 4 Triceps Stretches for Tight Muscles. Retrieved May 17, 2020, from https://www.healthline.com/health/exercise-fitness/tricep-stretches#stretches

REFERENCES

Elorreaga, N. (2018, February 4). Give Yourself A Full Body Mobility Assessment! –. Retrieved May 10, 2020, from https://www.nick-e.com/mobility-assessment/

Fischer-Colbrie, M. (2017, July 18). Stretching Improves Athletic Performance and Health. Retrieved May 17, 2020, from https://blog.bridgeathletic.com/stretching-improves-your-health-strength-training

Freutel, N. (2016, December 19). How to Perform a Lacrosse Ball Massage on Sore Muscles. Retrieved May 13, 2020, from https://www.healthline.com/health/fitness-exercise/lacrosse-ball-massage#3

For Care Education and Research (n.d). 15 Best back stretching exercises (with video). Retrieved May 13, 2020, from https://fcer.org/back-stretching-exercises/

Gelles, D. (n.d.). How to Meditate. Retrieved May 16, 2020, from https://www.nytimes.com/guides/well/how-to-meditate

Gupta, A. (2019, November 21). How to perform the Supine Spinal Twist to reduce lower back pain - watch video. Retrieved May 17, 2020, from https://www.timesnownews.com/health/article/how-to-perform-the-supine-spinal-twist-to-reduce-lower-back-pain-watch-video/517968

Hart Osteopathy. (n.d.). Is the Tension Between Your

REFERENCES

Shoulder Blades Difficult to Reach? This Stretch is for You! Retrieved May 17, 2020, from https://www.hartosteopathy.com/self-hug-stretch.html

Harvard Health Publishing. (2019, September 25). The importance of stretching. Retrieved May 10, 2020, from https://www.health.harvard.edu/staying-healthy/the-importance-of-stretching

Healthwise. (2019, June 26). Wrist: Exercises. Retrieved May 13, 2020, from https://myhealth.alberta.ca/Health/aftercareinformation/pages/conditions.aspx?hwid=ad1518

Jewell, T. (2019, July 5). Guide to Biohacking: Types, Safety, and How To. Retrieved May 17, 2020, from https://www.healthline.com/health/biohacking

Lackowski, R. (2016, June 24). Stretch of the Week: Seated Piriformis Stretch. Retrieved May 17, 2020, from https://www.athletico.com/2016/06/22/stretch-of-the-week-seated-piriformis-stretch/

Lindberg, S. (2020, March 11). Stretching: 9 Benefits, Plus Safety Tips and How to Start. Retrieved May 10, 2020, from https://www.healthline.com/health/benefits-of-stretching

Marin, K. (2015, March 13). The Importance of Breathing in Yoga. Retrieved May 16, 2020, from https://www.yogabhoga.com/blog/importance-breathing-yoga

Mateo, A. (2020, May 11). 4 Glute Stretches You Should Do Every Day to Run Faster and Avoid Injury. Retrieved May 13, 2020, from https://www.runnersworld.com/training/a28708481/glute-stretches/

McGee, K. (2014, May 12). 5 Health Benefits Of Child's Pose. Retrieved May 17, 2020, from https://www.doyou.com/5-health-benefits-of-childs-pose/

McGee, K. (2015, April 10). 25 Simple Ways to Balance Your Mind, Body, and Soul. Retrieved May 16, 2020, from https://www.doyou.com/25-simple-ways-to-balance-your-mind-body-and-soul-17694/

PhysioRoom. (2018, March 15). PhysioRoom's Guide to Foam Rollers. Retrieved May 13, 2020, from https://www.physioroom.com/info/physiorooms-guide-to-foam-rollers/

Physicians Diagnostics and Rehabilitation (n.d.). Cervical Spine Stretches. Retrieved May 13, 2020, from http://www.rosquistchiropractic.net/docs/SpineCarefortheTherapist.pdf

Popsugar Fitness. (2016, September 13). 5 Easy Ways to Stretch Your Calves. Retrieved May 17, 2020, from https://www.self.com/story/best-calf-stretches-running

Reed-Guy, B. L. M. A. L. (2020, February 3). Arthritis. Retrieved May 15, 2020, from https://www.healthline.com/health/arthritis#symptoms

REFERENCES

Rizopoulos, N. (2017, April 12). The Benefits of Pigeon Pose. Retrieved May 17, 2020, from https://www.yogajournal.com/lifestyle/hip-connections

Saint Luke's. (n.d.). Supine Hamstring Stretch. Retrieved May 14, 2020, from https://www.saintlukeskc.org/health-library/supine-hamstring-stretch

Seto, W. (2018, November 22). Neck, First Rib Pain & Stiffness: Anterior Scalene Muscle Stretch. Retrieved May 13, 2020, from https://insyncphysio.com/neck-first-rib-pain-stiffness-anterior-scalene-muscle-stretch/

Spotebi. (2017, July 4). Chest Stretch | Illustrated Exercise Guide. Retrieved May 17, 2020, from https://www.spotebi.com/exercise-guide/chest-stretch/

Stelter, G. (2016, December 18). 5 Good Yoga Stretches for Your Arms. Retrieved May 13, 2020, from https://www.healthline.com/health/fitness-exercise/arm-stretches#8

Stretch Relief. (2019, April 9). Is Stretching Good for My Mental Health? Retrieved May 16, 2020, from https://stretchrelief.com/stretching-good-for-mental-health/

Tran, P. (2015a, April 12). How to Do Sphinx Pose in Yoga. Retrieved May 13, 2020, from https://www.yogaoutlet.com/blogs/guides/how-to-do-sphinx-pose-in-yoga

Tran, P. (2015b, April 12). How to Do Wide-Legged

Standing Forward Fold in Yoga. Retrieved May 14, 2020, from https://www.yogaoutlet.com/blogs/guides/how-to-do-wide-legged-standing-forward-fold-in-yoga

Thielen, S. (2015, September 17). 5 Chest Stretch Variations. Retrieved May 13, 2020, from https://www.acefitness.org/education-and-resources/lifestyle/blog/5657/5-chest-stretch-variations/

UC Davis. (2014, April 29). Why Stretching is Extremely Important | Student Health and Counseling Services. Retrieved May 10, 2020, from https://shcs.ucdavis.edu/blog/archive/healthy-habits/why-stretching-extremely-important

Ultra Running. (2013, February 8). Benefits of Hamstring Stretches. Retrieved May 17, 2020, from https://www.ultrarunningltd.co.uk/training-schedule/stretching/benefits-of-hamstring-stretches

Winderl, A. C. M. (2018a, January 19). The 7 Best Stretches for Knee Pain. Retrieved May 13, 2020, from https://www.self.com/gallery/best-stretches-for-knee-pain

Winderl, A. C. M. (2018b, December 18). 12 Exercises and Stretches for Shoulder Pain. Retrieved May 13, 2020, from https://www.self.com/gallery/stretches-to-relieve-tight-shoulders

REFERENCES

Winderl, A. C. M. (2020, February 3). 12 Hip Stretches Your Body Really Needs. Retrieved May 13, 2020, from https://www.self.com/gallery/hip-stretches-your-body-really-needs-slideshow

Winderl, A. C. M. (2020, May 8). The 21 Best Stretching Exercises for Better Flexibility. Retrieved May 16, 2020, from https://www.self.com/gallery/essential-stretches-slideshow

Yoga Journal. (2017, April 12). Standing Forward Bend. Retrieved May 17, 2020, from https://www.yogajournal.com/poses/standing-forward-bend

Printed in Great Britain
by Amazon